A FEAST OF INFORMATION—
for people who love to eat but need to know the carbohydrate count of their meals.

THE BARBARA KRAUS 1983 CARBOHYDRATE GUIDE TO BRAND NAMES & BASIC FOODS lists thousands of basic and ready-to-eat foods from appetizers to desserts—carry it to the supermarket, to the restaurant, to the beach, to the coffee cart, and on trips.

Flip through these fact-filled pages. Mix, match, and keep track of grams as they add up. But remember, strawberry shortcake is fattening any way you slice it!

The Barbara Kraus
1983 Carbohydrate
Guide to
Brand Names and
Basic Foods

SIGNET Books for Your Reference Shelf

(0451)

☐ **THE LOS ANGELES TIMES NATURAL FOOD COOKBOOK by Jeanne Voltz, Food Editor, Women's Day Magazine.** Discover the joys of cooking and eating naturally with this book of over 600 savory, simple-to-follow recipes. Whether you are concerned with taste or nutrition, these delicious and healthy recipes—high in fiber content—will delight everyone from the gourmet chef to the dedicated dieter. (112377—$2.95)

☐ **CALORIES AND CARBOHYDRATES by Barbara Kraus.** Foreword by Edward B. Greenspan, M.D. Revised edition. This dictionary contains 8,000 brand names and basic foods with their caloric and carbohydrate counts. Recommended by doctors, nutritionists, and family food planners as an indispensable aid to those who must be concerned with what they eat, it will become the most important diet reference source you will ever own. (097742—$3.50)*

☐ **THE JEWISH LOW-CHOLESTEROL COOKBOOK by Roberta Leviton, with an introduction by Rabbi Meyer J. Strassfeld.** This modern, health-conscious cookbook offers over 200 taste-tempting recipes from around the world to help you cut your cholesterol and lose weight without sacrificing any of those traditional favorites. (086236—$2.50)

☐ **LIVING SALT FREE . . . AND EASY by Anna Houston Thorburn with Phyllis Turner.** The first specific guide to medically approved low sodium foods for those who want to live to eat as well as eat to live. Includes a sizable collection of recipes that tastes too good to be diet food! (071204—$1.50)

☐ **GOURMET COOKING BY THE CLOCK by William and Chesbrough Rayner.** Here at last are full instructions to one of the fine points of cooking . . . the art of perfect timing. These are easy-to-follow recipes for everything from appetizers to desserts with each step of preparation and cooking timed by the clock. (090446—$1.95)

*Price slightly higher in Canada

The Barbara Kraus 1983 Carbohydrate Guide to Brand Names and Basic Foods

••••——◆——••••

Ø

A SIGNET BOOK

NEW AMERICAN LIBRARY

TIMES MIRROR

*For Mickey, Marge, Esther and
Jean Cavagnaro*

NAL BOOKS ARE AVAILABLE AT QUANTITY DISCOUNTS
WHEN USED TO PROMOTE PRODUCTS OR SERVICES. FOR
INFORMATION PLEASE WRITE TO PREMIUM MARKETING DIVISION,
THE NEW AMERICAN LIBRARY, INC., 1633 BROADWAY,
NEW YORK, NEW YORK 10019.

Excerpted from *Dictionary of Calories and Carbohydrates*

SIGNET TRADEMARK REG. U.S. PAT. OFF. AND FOREIGN COUNTRIES
REGISTERED TRADEMARK—MARCA REGISTRADA
HECHO EN CHICAGO, U.S.A.

SIGNET, SIGNET CLASSICS, MENTOR, PLUME, MERIDIAN AND NAL
BOOKS *are published by The New American Library, Inc.,
1633 Broadway, New York, New York 10019*

FIRST PRINTING, JANUARY, 1983

1 2 3 4 5 6 7 8 9

PRINTED IN THE UNITED STATES OF AMERICA

Foreword

The composition of the foods we eat is not static: it changes from time to time. In the case of *brand-name* products, manufacturers alter their recipes to reflect the availability of ingredients, advances in technology, or improvements in formulae. Each year new products appear on the market and some old ones are discontinued.

On the other hand, information on *basic foods* such as meats, vegetables, and fruits may also change as a result of the development of better analytical methods, different growing conditions, or new marketing practices. These changes, however, are usually relatively small as compared with those in manufactured products.

Some differences may be found between the values in this book and those appearing on the product labels. This is usually due to the fact that the Food and Drug Administration permits manufacturers to round the figures reported on labels. The data in this book are reported as calculated without rounding. If large differences between the two sets of values are noted, they may be due to changes in product formulae, and in those cases the label data should be used.

For all these reasons, a book of carbohydrate or nutritive values of foods must be kept up to date by a periodic reviewing and revision of the data presented.

Therefore, this handy carbohydrate counter will provide each year the most current and accurate estimates available. Generous use of this little book will help you and your family to select the right foods and the proper number of carbohydrates each member requires.

Good eating in 1983! For 1984, we'll pick up the new products, drop any has-beens, and make whatever other changes are necessary.

Barbara Kraus

Why This Book?

Some of the data presented here can be found in more detail in my best-selling *Calories and Carbohydrates,* a dictionary of 8,000 brand names and basic foods. Complete as it is, it is meant to be used as a reference book at home or in the office and not to be squeezed into a suit jacket or evening bag—it's just too big.

Therefore, responding to the need for a portable carbohydrate guide, and one which can reflect food changes often, I have written this smaller and handier version. The selection of material and the additional new entries provide readers with pertinent data on thousands of products that they would prepare at home to take to work, eat in a restaurant or luncheonette, nibble on from the coffee cart, take to the beach, buy in the candy store, etcetera.

For the sake of saving space and providing you with a greater selection of products, I had to make certain compromises: whereas in the giant book there are several physical descriptions of a product, here there is but one.

What Are Carbohydrates?

Carbohydrates—which include sugars, starches, and acids —are one of several chemical compounds in food which yield calories. Their main function is to supply energy to body cells, particularly muscle and brain cells. The amount of carbohydrates varies from zero in meats, fish, and poultry, to heavy concentrations in such foods as syrups, cereals, bread, beans, some fresh and all dried fruit, and root vegetables, such as potatoes.

As of this date, the most respected nutritional researchers insist that some carbohydrate is necessary every day for maintaining good health. The amount to be included is an individual matter, and in any drastic effort to alter your eating patterns, be sure to consult your doctor first.

ABBREVIATIONS AND SYMBOLS

* = prepared as package directs[1]
< = less than
& = and
" = inch
canned = bottles or jars as well as cans
dia. = diameter
fl. = fluid
liq. = liquid
lb. = pound
med. = medium

oz. = ounce
pkg. = package
pt. = pint
qt. = quart
sq. = square
T. = tablespoon
Tr. = trace
tsp. = teaspoon
wt. = weight

Italics or name in parentheses = registered trademark, ®. All data not identified by company or trademark are based on material obtained from the United States Department of Agriculture or Health, Education and Welfare/Food and Agriculture Organization.

EQUIVALENTS

By Weight
1 pound = 16 ounces
1 ounce = 28.35 grams
3.52 ounces = 100 grams

By Volume
1 quart = 4 cups
1 cup = 8 fluid ounces
1 cup = ½ pint
1 cup = 16 tablespoons
2 tablespoons = 1 fluid ounce
1 tablespoon = 3 teaspoons
1 pound butter = 4 sticks or 2 cups

[1] If the package directions call for whole or skim milk, the data given here are for whole milk unless otherwise stated.

Food and Description	Measure or Quantity	Carbohydrates (grams)

A

Food and Description	Measure or Quantity	Carbohydrates (grams)
ABALONE, canned	4-oz.	2.6
ABISANTE LIQUEUR (Leroux)	1 fl. oz.	1.0
AC'CENT	¼ tsp.	0.
ALEXANDER COCKTAIL MIX (Holland House)	1 serving	16.0
ALLSPICE (French's)	1 tsp.	1.3
ALMOND:		
In shell	10 nuts	2.0
Shelled, raw, natural with skins	1 oz.	5.5
Roasted, dry (Planters)	1 oz.	6.0
Roasted, oil (Fisher)	1 oz.	5.5
ALMOND EXTRACT (Virginia Dare) 34% alcohol	1 tsp.	0.
ALPHA-BITS, cereal (Post)	1 cup	23.8
AMARETTO DELIGHT COCKTAIL, canned (Mr. Boston)	3 fl. oz.	27.6
AMARETTO DI SARONNO	1 fl. oz.	9.0
AMARETTO SOUR COCKTAIL, canned (Mr. Boston)	3 fl. oz.	15.6
A.M. FRUIT DRINK (Mott's)	6 fl. oz.	22.0
ANCHOVY, PICKLED, canned, flat or rolled, not heavily salted, drained	2-oz. can	.1
ANISETTE LIQUEUR (Mr. Boston)	1 fl. oz.	10.8
APPLE:		
Eaten with skin	2½″ dia.	15.3
Eaten without skin	2½″ dia.	13.9
Canned:		
(Del Monte) dried	1 cup	37.2
(Comstock):		
Rings, drained	1 ring	7.0
Sliced	⅛ of 21-oz. can	10.0
(Sun-Maid) dried	2-oz. serving	40.0
Frozen, sweetened	10-oz. pkg.	68.9
APPLE BROWN BETTY	1 cup	63.9
APPLE BUTTER (Smucker's) cider	1 T.	9.0
APPLE-CHERRY JUICE COCKTAIL, canned *Musselman's*	8 fl. oz.	28.0
APPLE CIDER:		
Canned (Mott's) sweet	½ cup	14.6
*Mix, Country Time	8 fl. oz.	24.5
APPLE-CRANBERRY DRINK (Hi-C):		
Canned	6 fl. oz.	21.0

1

Food and Description	Measure or Quantity	Carbohydrates (grams)
*Mix	6 fl. oz.	18.0
APPLE-CRANBERRY JUICE,		
canned (Lincoln)	6 fl. oz.	26.0
APPLE DRINK:		
Canned:		
Capri Sun, natural	6¾ fl. oz.	22.7
(Hi-C)	6 fl. oz.	23.0
*Mix (Hi-C)	6 fl. oz.	18.0
APPLE DUMPLING, frozen		
(Pepperidge Farm)	1 dumpling	31.0
APPLE, ESCALLOPED, frozen		
(Stouffer's)	4-oz. serving	27.8
APPLE-GRAPE JUICE, canned:		
Musselman's	6 fl. oz.	21.0
(Red Cheek)	6 fl. oz.	22.6
APPLE JACKS, cereal(Kellogg's)	1 cup	26.0
APPLE JAM (Smucker's)	1 T.	13.5
APPLE JELLY:		
Sweetened (Smucker's)	1 T.	14.0
Dietetic (See APPLE SPREAD)		
APPLE JUICE:		
Canned:		
(Lincoln's) cocktail	6 fl. oz.	24.7
(Minute Maid)	6 fl. oz.	24.0
(Mott's)	6 fl. oz.	19.0
Musselman's	6 fl. oz.	21.0
(Red Cheek)	6 fl. oz.	21.2
(Seneca Foods) Vitamin C	6 fl. oz.	22.0
Chilled (Minute Maid)	6 fl. oz.	24.0
*Frozen:		
(Minute Maid)	6 fl. oz.	24.0
(Seneca Foods) Vitamin C	6 fl. oz.	22.0
APPLE PIE (See PIE, Apple)		
APPLE SAUCE:		
Canned, regular pack:		
(Del Monte)	½ cup	23.6
(Mott's):		
Natural	4-oz. serving	27.5
With ground cranberries	4-oz. serving	27.0
Musselman's	½ cup	23.5
Canned, dietetic:		
(Diet Delight)	½ cup	13.0
(Featherweight) water pack	½ cup	12.0
(Mott's) natural	4-oz. serving	11.0
Musselman's, natural	½ cup	12.0
(Seneca Foods) 100% natural	½ cup	12.0
(S&W) *Nutradiet*, water pack	½ cup	14.0

Food and Description	Measure or Quantity	Carbohydrates (grams)
APPLE SPREAD, low sugar:		
(Dia-Mel)	1 T.	0.
(Diet Delight)	1 T.	3.0
(Featherweight):		
Regular	1 T.	4.0
Artificially sweetened	1 T.	1.0
(Slenderella)	1 T.	6.0
(Smucker's)	1 T.	6.0
(Tillie Lewis) *Tasti Diet*	1 T.	3.0
APRICOT:		
Fresh, whole	1 apricot	4.5
Canned, regular pack:		
(Del Monte) whole, peeled	1 cup	50.0
(Libby's) halves, heavy syrup	1 cup	53.6
(Stokely-Van Camp)		
solids & liq.	1 cup	54.0
Canned, dietetic pack:		
(Del Monte) *Lite*, syrup pack	½ cup	15.1
(Diet Delight):		
Syrup pack	½ cup	15.0
Water pack	½ cup	9.0
(Featherweight):		
Juice pack	½ cup	12.0
Water pack	½ cup	9.0
(S&W) *Nutradiet*, solids & liq.:		
Halves, juice pack	½ cup	13.0
Halves, water pack	½ cup	9.0
Whole, juice pack	½ cup	10.0
Dried:		
(Del Monte)	½ cup	39.9
(Sun-Maid; Sunsweet)	¼ cup	30.0
APRICOT LIQUEUR (DeKuyper)	1 fl. oz.	8.3
APRICOT NECTAR, canned (Del Monte)	½ cup	18.0
APRICOT-PINEAPPLE NECTAR, canned, dietetic (S&W) *Nutradiet*	6 fl. oz.	12.0
APRICOT & PINEAPPLE PRESERVE OR JAM:		
Sweetened (Smucker's)	1 T.	13.5
Dietetic (See APRICOT & PINEAPPLE SPREAD)		
APRICOT & PINEAPPLE SPREAD, low sugar:		
(Diet Delight)	1 T.	3.0
(Featherweight) artificially sweetened	1 T.	1.0

Food and Description	Measure or Quantity	Carbohydrates (grams)
(S&W) *Nutradiet*	1 T.	3.0
(Tillie Lewis) *Tasti-Diet*	1 T.	2.8
APRICOT PRESERVE OR JAM:		
Sweetened (Smucker's)	1 T.	13.5
Dietetic:		
(Dia-Mel)	1 T.	0.
(Featherweight)	1 T.	4.0
APRICOT SOUR COCKTAIL,		
canned (National Distillers) *Duet*, 12½% alcohol	2 fl. oz.	1.6
AQUAVIT (Leroux)	1 fl. oz.	Tr.
ARTICHOKE:		
Boiled	12-oz. artichoke	42.1
Canned (Cara Mia) marinated, drained	6-oz. jar	12.6
Frozen:		
(Birds Eye)	⅓ of pkg.	5.5
(Cara Mia)	⅓ of pkg.	7.5
ASPARAGUS:		
Boiled	1 spear (½" dia. at base)	.7
Canned, regular pack, spears, solids & liq.:		
(Del Monte) green or white	1 cup	6.4
(Festal) green	1 cup	6.4
(Festal) white	1 cup	7.4
(Green Giant) green	½ of 10½-oz. can	2.5
(Stokely-Van Camp)	1 cup	6.0
Canned, dietetic pack, solids & liq.:		
(Diet Delight)	½ cup	2.0
(Featherweight) cut spears	½ cup	3.0
(S&W) *Nutradiet*, spears	½ cup	4.0
Frozen:		
(Birds Eye) cuts	⅓ of pkg.	3.0
(Green Giant) cuts, butter sauce	1 cup	7.0
(McKenzie Seabrook Farms)	⅓ of pkg.	3.8
(Stouffer's) souffle	⅓ of pkg.	8.0
*ASPARAGUS SOUP (Campbell) cream of	10-oz. serving	12.0
ASTI WINE (Gancia)	3 fl. oz.	18.0
AVOCADO, all varieties	1 fruit	14.3
*AWAKE (Birds Eye)	6 fl. oz.	21.2
AYDS:		
Butterscotch	1 piece	5.7

4

Food and Description	Measure or Quantity	Carbohydrates (grams)
Vanilla, chocolate or chocolate mint	1 piece	5.5

B

Food and Description	Measure or Quantity	Carbohydrates (grams)
BACON, broiled (Oscar Mayer):		
Regular slice	6-gram slice	.1
Thick slice	11-gram slice	.2
BACON BITS:		
(Betty Crocker) *Bac*Os*	1 T.	2.0
(Durkee) imitation	1 tsp.	.5
(French's) imitation	1 tsp.	Tr.
(Hormel)	1 tsp.	.1
(Oscar Mayer) real	1 tsp.	.1
BACON, CANADIAN, unheated:		
(Hormel) sliced	1-oz. serving	.1
(Oscar Mayer) 93% fat free	1-oz. slice	0.
BACON, SIMULATED, cooked:		
(Oscar Mayer) *Lean 'N Tasty*, beef or pork	1 slice	.2
(Swift) *Sizzlean*	1 slice	0.
BAGEL (Lender's) garlic, onion or poppyseed	2-oz. bagel	31.5
BAKING POWDER (Calumet)	1 tsp.	1.0
BAMBOO SHOOTS:		
Raw, trimmed	¼ lb.	5.9
Canned, drained:		
(Chun King)	½ of 8½-oz. can	2.0
(La Choy)	½ cup	2.2
BANANA, unpeeled, medium	6.2-oz. banana	26.4
BARBECUE SEASONING (French's)	1 tsp.	1.0
BARDOLINO WINE (Antinori)	1 fl. oz.	6.3
BARLEY, pearled (Quaker Scotch)	¼ cup	36.3
***BARLEY & MUSHROOM SOUP,** frozen (Mother's Own)	8-oz. serving	8.0
BASIL (French's)	1 tsp.	.7
BASS:		
Baked, stuffed	3½" x 4½" x 1½"	23.4
Oven-fried	8¾" x 4½" x ⅝"	13.4
BAY LEAF (French's)	1 tsp.	1.0
B & B LIQUEUR	1 fl. oz.	5.7
B.B.Q. SAUCE & BEEF, frozen (Banquet) *Cookin' Bag*, sliced	5-oz. cooking bag	12.5
BEAN, BAKED, canned:		
With pork & molasses sauce	1 cup	53.8

Food and Description	Measure or Quantity	Carbohydrates (grams)
With pork & tomato sauce (Ann Page):	1 cup	48.5
With pork & molasses sauce, Boston style	8-oz. serving	49.8
With pork & tomato sauce (B&M):	8-oz. serving	41.6
Pea bean with pork in brown sugar sauce	8-oz. can	49.0
Red kidney bean in brown sugar sauce	8-oz. serving	50.0
Yellow eye bean in brown sugar sauce (Campbell)	8-oz. serving	50.0
Home style	8-oz. can	52.0
With pork in tomato sauce	8-oz. can	44.0
(Grandma Brown's)	8-oz. serving	54.1
(Libby's) Deep Brown:		
With pork & molasses sauce	7-oz. serving	40.6
Vegetarian in tomato sauce	7-oz. serving	40.8
(Sultana) with pork & tomato sauce	8-oz. serving	41.8
(Van Camp):		
With brown sugar sauce	1 cup	61.0
With pork	1 cup	47.0
Vegetarian style	1 cup	48.0
BEAN, BLACK, dry	1 cup	122.4
BEAN & FRANKFURTER, canned (Campbell) in tomato and molasses sauce	8-oz. can	43.2
(Hormel) Short Orders, 'N Wiener	7½-oz. can	29.0
BEAN & FRANKFURTER DINNER, frozen:		
(Banquet)	10¾-oz. dinner	63.1
(Morton)	10¾-oz. dinner	79.4
(Swanson) TV Brand	11¼-oz. dinner	75.0
BEAN, GARBANZO, canned, dietetic (S&W) Nutradiet	½ cup	19.0
BEAN, GREEN:		
Boiled, 1½" to 2" pieces, drained	½ cup	3.7
Canned, regular pack:		
(Comstock) solids & liq.	½ cup	4.0
(Del Monte) French, drained	½ cup	4.9
(Festal) cut, drained	½ cup	5.3
(Green Giant) French or whole, solids & liq.	½ cup	2.6
(Kounty Kist) French, solids & liq.	½ cup	2.6

Food and Description	Measure or Quantity	Carbohydrates (grams)
(Libby's)		
Cut, solids & liq.	½ cup	4.1
French style, solids & liq.	½ cup	4.2
(Stokely-Van Camp) solids & liq.	½ cup	3.5
(Sunshine) solids & liq.	½ cup	3.8
Canned, dietetic pack:		
(Diet Delight) solids & liq.	½ cup	3.0
(Featherweight) solids & liq.	½ cup	5.0
(S&W) *Nutradiet*	½ cup	4.0
Frozen:		
(Birds Eye):		
Cut	⅓ of pkg.	5.0
With toasted almonds	⅓ of pkg.	7.8
(Green Giant):		
Butter sauce	⅓ of pkg.	3.0
Mushroom sauce	⅓ of pkg.	6.1
(McKenzie Seabrook Farms)	⅓ of pkg.	5.8
(Southland) cut or French style	⅕ of 16-oz. pkg.	5.0
BEAN, GREEN, & MUSHROOM CASSEROLE, frozen (Stouffer's)	½ of pkg.	11.9
BEAN, GREEN WITH POTATOES, canned (Sunshine) sloids & liq.	½ cup	7.0
BEAN, GREEN, PUREE, canned, dietetic (Featherweight)	1 cup	15.0
BEAN, ITALIAN:		
Canned (Del Monte) drained	½ cup	8.2
Frozen (Seabrook Farms)	⅓ of pkg.	7.1
BEAN, KIDNEY:		
Canned, regular pack:		
(Furman) red, fancy, light	½ cup	21.2
(Van Camp) red	1 cup	38.0
Canned, dietetic (S&W) *Nutradiet* solids & liq.	½ cup	16.0
BEAN, LIMA:		
Boiled, drained	½ cup	16.8
Canned, regular pack:		
(Del Monte) drained	½ cup	19.7
(Libby's) solids & liq.	½ cup	16.0
(Sultana) baby	¼ of 15-oz. can	12.0
(Sultana) butter bean	¼ of 15-oz. can	14.6
Canned, dietetic pack (Featherweight) solids & liq.	½ cup	16.0
Frozen:		
(Birds Eye):		
Baby limas	⅓ of pkg.	22.0

Food and Description	Measure or Quantity	Carbohydrates (grams)
Fordhooks	⅓ of pkg.	18.0
(Green Giant):		
Baby limas	¼ of pkg.	22.4
Speckled butter beans, Southern recipe	⅓ of pkg.	13.2
(McKenzie) baby limas	⅓ of pkg.	23.6
(Seabrook Farms):		
Baby limas	⅓ of pkg.	23.6
Baby butter bean	⅓ of pkg.	26.1
Fordhooks	⅓ of pkg.	17.9
BEAN, PINTO (Del Monte) spicy	½ cup	19.0
BEAN, RED MEXICAN (Green Giant)	¼ of 15½-oz. can	17.5
BEAN, REFRIED:		
(Del Monte) regular or spicy	½ cup	20.0
Old El Paso	½ of 8¼-oz. can	17.5
(Ortega)	½ cup	25.0
BEAN SALAD:		
(Green Giant)	4½-oz. serving	19.9
(Nalley's)	4½-oz. serving	29.4
BEAN SOUP:		
*(Ann Page) condensed, with bacon	1 cup	19.0
(Campbell):		
Chunky, with ham, old fashioned	11-oz. can	35.0
*Condensed:		
With bacon	11-oz. serving	29.0
Semi-condensed, *Soup For One*, old fashioned with ham	11-oz. serving	31.0
(Grandma Brown's)	8-oz. serving	29.1
BEAN SOUP, BLACK (Crosse & Blackwell) with sherry	13-oz. can	36.0
BEAN SPROUT:		
Fresh:		
Mung, raw	½ lb.	15.0
Mung, boiled, drained	¼ lb.	5.9
Soy, raw	½ lb.	12.0
Soy, boiled, drained	¼ lb.	4.2
Canned:		
(Chun King) drained	8-oz. serving	5.9
(La Choy) drained	⅔ cup	.9
BEAN, WHITE, Great Northern, cooked	½ cup	18.0
BEAN, YELLOW OR WAX:		
Boiled, 1″ pieces, drained	½ cup	5.2

Food and Description	Measure or Quantity	Carbohydrates (grams)
Canned, regular pack:		
(Comstock) solids & liq.	½ cup	4.5
(Del Monte) cut, solids & liq.	½ cup	3.4
(Festal) cut or French style, solids & liq.	½ cup	3.4
(Libby's) cut, solids & liq.	4-oz. serving	4.4
(Stokely-Van Camp) solids & liq.	½ cup	4.0
Canned, dietetic pack		
(Featherweight) cut	½ cup	5.0
Frozen (Birds Eye) cut	⅓ of pkg.	4.0
BEEF	Any quantity	0.
BEEFAMATO COCKTAIL (Mott's)	6 fl. oz.	15.0
BEEF BOUILLON, *MBT*	1 packet	2.0
BEEF, CHIPPED:		
Cooked, home recipe	½ cup	8.7
Frozen, creamed:		
(Banquet) *Cookin' Bag*	5-oz. pkg.	10.5
(Stouffer's)	5½-oz. serving	10.0
(Swanson)	10½-oz. entree	15.0
BEEF DINNER OR ENTREE, frozen:		
(Banquet):		
Regular	11-oz. dinner	20.9
Chopped	11-oz. dinner	32.8
Man Pleaser, sliced	20-oz. dinner	63.7
(Morton):		
Regular	10-oz. dinner	20.0
Country Table, sliced	14-oz. dinner	55.7
Steak House, sirloin strip	9½-oz. dinner	45.2
Steak House, tenderloin	9½-oz. dinner	43.2
(Swanson):		
Hungry Man, chopped	18-oz. dinner	70.0
Hungry Man, sliced	17-oz. dinner	51.0
Hungry Man, sliced	12½-oz. entree	23.0
TV Brand	11½-oz. dinner	34.0
TV Brand, chopped sirloin	10-oz. dinner	36.0
3-course	15-oz. dinner	57.0
(Weight Watchers):		
Beefsteak, 2-compartment meal	9¾-oz. pkg.	12.0
Sirloin in mushroom sauce, 3-compartment meal	13-oz. pkg.	16.0
BEEF, DRIED, canned:		
(Hormel) *Short Orders*	7½-oz. can	9.0
(Swift)	1-oz. serving	0.
BEEF GOULASH (Hormel) *Short Orders*	7½-oz. can	16.0

9

Food and Description	Measure or Quantity	Carbohydrates (grams)
BEEF, GROUND, SEASONING MIX:		
*(Durkee):		
Regular	1 cup	9.0
With onion	1 cup	6.5
(French's) with onion	¼ of 1⅛-oz. pkg.	6.0
BEEF HASH, ROAST:		
Canned, *Mary Kitchen:*		
Regular	7½-oz. serving	17.9
Short Orders	7½-oz. can	19.0
Frozen (Stouffer's)	5¾-oz. serving	10.9
BEEF PEPPER ORIENTAL:		
*Canned (La Choy):		
Regular	¾ cup	8.0
Bi-pack	¾ cup	12.0
Frozen (Chun King):		
Dinner	11-oz. dinner	43.0
Pouch	6-oz. serving	10.0
BEEF PIE, frozen:		
(Banquet)	8-oz. pie	40.9
(Morton)	8-oz. pie	31.8
(Stouffer's)	10-oz. pie	37.8
(Swanson):		
Regular	8-oz. pie	44.0
Hungry Man	16-oz. pie	65.0
Hungry Man, steak burger	16-oz. pie	69.0
BEEF PUFFS, frozen (Durkee)	1 piece	3.0
BEEF SHORT RIBS, frozen (Stouffer's) boneless, with vegetable gravy	5¾-oz. serving	2.0
BEEF SOUP:		
Canned, regular pack:		
(Campbell):		
Chunky:		
Regular	10¾-oz. can	23.0
With noodles	10¾-oz. can	29.0
*Condensed:		
Regular	11-oz. serving	15.0
Broth	10-oz. serving	2.0
Broth & barley	10-oz. serving	13.0
Broth & noodles	10-oz. serving	10.0
Consomme	10-oz. serving	2.0
Mushroom	10-oz. serving	8.0
Noodle	10-oz. serving	9.0
(College Inn) broth	1 cup	1.0
(Swanson) broth	½ of 13¾-oz. can	1.0
*Canned, dietetic pack (Dia-Mel) & noodle	8-oz. serving	5.0

Food and Description	Measure or Quantity	Carbohydrates (grams)
BEEF SOUP MIX:		
Carmel Kosher	6 fl. oz.	1.8
(Lipton) Cup-A-Soup:		
Regular, & noodle		8.0
Lots-A-Noodles		21.0
BEEF SPREAD, ROAST, canned		
(Underwood)	½ of 4¾-oz. can	Tr.
BEEF STEAK, BREADED, frozen		
(Hormel)	4-oz. serving	12.7
BEEF STEW:		
Home recipe, made with lean beef chuck	1 cup	15.2
Canned, regular pack:		
Dinty Moore:		
Regular	7½-oz. serving	12.8
Short Orders	7½-oz. can	14.0
(Libby's)	1 cup	33.8
(Morton House)	⅓ of 24-oz. can	17.0
(Nalley's)	7½-oz. serving	17.0
(Swanson)	7½-oz. serving	18.0
Canned, dietetic pack:		
(Dia-Mel)	8-oz. can	19.0
(Featherweight)	7¼-oz. can	24.0
Frozen:		
(Green Giant) & biscuits, Bake 'n Serve	14-oz. pkg.	40.6
(Stouffer's)	10-oz. serving	15.9
BEEF STEW SEASONING MIX:		
*(Durkee)	1 cup	16.7
(French's)	1⅛-oz. pkg.	30.0
BEEF STIX (Vienna)	1-oz. serving	1.4
BEEF STROGANOFF, frozen		
(Stouffer's)	9¾-oz. serving	30.7
***BEEF STROGANOFF**		
SEASONING MIX (Durkee)	1 cup	71.2
BEER & ALE:		
Regular:		
Black Horse Ale	8 fl. oz.	9.2
Black Label	8 fl. oz.	7.5
Budweiser	8 fl. oz.	8.9
Busch Bavarian	8 fl. oz.	8.0
Heidelberg	8 fl. oz.	7.1
Knickerbocker	8 fl. oz.	9.1
Meister Brau Premium, regular or draft	8 fl. oz.	7.3
Michelob	8 fl. oz.	11.0

11

Food and Description	Measure or Quantity	Carbohydrates (grams)
North Star, regular	8 fl. oz.	9.9
Pearl Premium	8 fl. oz.	8.3
Pfeifer, regular	8 fl. oz.	9.9
Pfeifer, 3.2 low gravity	8 fl. oz.	9.1
Red Cap	8 fl. oz.	7.2
Rheingold	8 fl. oz.	9.1
Schmidt, regular	8 fl. oz.	9.9
Schmidt, 3.2 low gravity	8 fl. oz.	9.1
Stag	8 fl. oz.	7.5
Stroh Bohemian, regular	8 fl. oz.	9.1
Stroh Bohemian, 3.2 low gravity	8 fl. oz.	7.7
Tuborg, USA	8 fl. oz.	8.1
Light or low carbohydrate:		
Budweiser Light	8 fl. oz.	4.0
Gablinger's	8 fl. oz.	.1
Meister Brau Lite	8 fl. oz.	.9
Michelob Light	8 fl. oz.	8.0
Natural Light	8 fl. oz.	4.0
Pearl Light	8 fl. oz.	1.0
Stroh Light	8 fl. oz.	4.7
BEER, NEAR:		
Goetz Pale	8 fl. oz.	2.6
Kingsbury (Heileman)	8 fl. oz.	7.1
(Metbrew)	8 fl. oz.	9.1
BEET:		
Boiled, whole	2″ dia. beet	3.6
Boiled, sliced	½ cup	7.3
Canned, regular pack:		
(Del Monte):		
Pickled, solids & liq.	½ cup	18.1
Sliced, solids & liq.	½ cup	7.0
(Greenwood):		
Harvard, solids & liq.	½ cup	16.0
Pickled, solids & liq.	½ cup	27.5
(Libby's) Harvard, solids & liq.	½ cup	20.8
(Stokely-Van Camp) Pickled, solids & liq.	½ cup	22.5
Canned, dietetic pack, solids & liq.		
(Blue Boy) whole	4-oz. serving	9.2
(Comstock) water pack	½ cup	6.5
(Featherweight)	½ cup	10.0
(S&W) *Nutradiet*	½ cup	9.0
BEET PUREE, canned, dietetic (Featherweight)	1 cup	20.0
BENEDICTINE LIQUEUR (Julius Wile)	1½ fl. oz.	15.5
BIG H, burger sauce (Hellmann's)	1 T.	1.6

Food and Description	Measure or Quantity	Carbohydrates (grams)
BIG MAC (See McDONALD'S)		
BIG WHEEL (Hostess)	1 cake	21.5
BISCUIT DOUGH, refrigerated (Pillsbury):		
Baking Powder, *1869 Brand*	1 biscuit	13.5
Big Country	1 biscuit	15.5
Big Country, good 'n buttery	1 biscuit	14.0
Buttermilk:		
Regular	1 biscuit	10.0
1869 Brand	1 biscuit	13.5
Extra Lights	1 biscuit	10.5
Hungry Jack, flaky	1 biscuit	13.0
Butter Tastin, Hungry Jack	1 biscuit	11.0
Country style	1 biscuit	10.0
Dinner	1 biscuit	7.5
Oven Ready, Ballard	1 biscuit	9.5
Prize	1 biscuit	9.5
BITTERS (Angostura)	1 tsp.	2.0
BLACKBERRY, fresh, hulled	1 cup	18.8
BLACKBERRY JELLY:		
Sweetened (Smucker's)	1 T.	13.5
Dietetic (See BLACKBERRY SPREAD)		
BLACKBERRY LIQUEUR (Bols)	1 fl. oz.	12.8
BLACKBERRY PRESERVE OR JAM:		
Sweetened (Smucker's)	1 T.	13.7
Dietetic:		
(Dia-Mel)	1 T.	0.
(Diet Delight)	1 T.	3.3
(Featherweight)	1 T.	4.0
(S&W) *Nutradiet*	1 T.	3.0
BLACKBERRY SPREAD, low sugar:		
(Diet Delight)	1 T.	3.0
(Featherweight)	1 T.	4.0
(Slenderella)	1 T.	6.0
(Smucker's)	1 T.	6.0
BLACKBERRY WINE (Mogen David)	3 fl. oz.	18.7
BLACK-EYED PEAS:		
Canned:		
(Sultana) with pork	7½-oz. serving	33.9
(Sunshine) with pork, solids & liq.	½ cup	16.1
Frozen:		
(Birds Eye)	⅓ of pkg.	23.0
(Green Giant)	⅓ of pkg.	12.7
(McKenzie)	⅓ of pkg.	22.7

13

Food and Description	Measure or Quantity	Carbohydrates (grams)
(Seabrook Farms)	⅛ of pkg.	22.7
(Southland)	⅙ of 16-oz. pkg.	21.0
BLACK RUSSIAN COCKTAIL MIX		
(Holland House)	1½ fl. oz.	34.5
BLINTZE, frozen (King Kold)		
cheese	2½-oz. piece	21.4
BLOODY MARY MIX:		
Dry (Bar-Tender's)	1 serving	5.7
Liquid (Sacramento)	5½-fl.-oz. can	9.1
BLUEBERRY, fresh	½ cup	11.2
BLUEBERRY PIE (See PIE, Blueberry)		
BLUEBERRY PRESERVE OR JAM:		
Sweetened (Smucker's)	1 T.	13.7
Dietetic (Dia-Mel)	1 T.	0.
BLUEFISH, broiled	1½″ x 3″ x ½″ piece	0.
BODY BUDDIES, cereal (General Mills)	1 oz.	25.0
BOLOGNA:		
(Best's Kosher; Oscherwitz)		
Chub	1-oz. serving	1.0
Sliced	1-oz. serving	1.0
(Eckrich):		
Beef, garlic, pickled, ring or sliced	1-oz. serving	1.5
Sliced thick	1.7-oz. slice	3.0
(Hormel):		
Beef	1-oz. slice	.3
Coarse ground, ring	1-oz. serving	.9
Fine ground, ring	1-oz. serving	.6
Meat	1-oz. slice	.2
(Oscar Mayer):		
Beef	.5-oz. slice	.4
Beef	1-oz. slice	.8
Beef	1.3-oz. slice	1.1
Beef Lebanon	.8-oz. slice	.4
Meat	.5-oz. slice	.3
Meat	1-oz. slice	.5
(Swift)	1-oz. slice	1.5
(Vienna) beef	1-oz. serving	.7
BOLOGNA & CHEESE (Oscar Mayer)	.8-oz. slice	.6
BONITO, canned (Star-Kist)	Any quantity	0.
BOO*BERRY, cereal (General Mills)	1 cup	24.0
BORSCHT, canned:		
Regular:		
Gold's)	8-oz. serving	17.5
(Mother's) old fashioned	8-oz. serving	21.3

14

Food and Description	Measure or Quantity	Carbohydrates (grams)
Dietetic or low calorie:		
(Gold's)	8-oz. serving	17.5
(Mother's):		
Artificially sweetened	8-oz. serving	6.1
Unsalted	8-oz. serving	25.1
(Rokeach)	8-oz. serving	6.7
BOSCO (See SYRUP)		
BOWL O' NOODLES (Nestlé) any flavor	1½-oz. envelope	29.0
BOYSENBERRY JELLY		
(Smucker's)	1 T.	13.5
BOYSENBERRY PRESERVE OR JAM:		
Sweetened (Smucker's)	1 T.	13.5
Dietetic:		
(Slenderella)	1 T.	6.0
(S&W) *Nutradiet*	1 T.	3.0
BOYSENBERRY SPREAD, imitation (Smucker's)	1 T.	6.0
BRAN, crude	1 oz.	17.5
BRAN BREAKFAST CEREAL:		
(Crawford's) & dates	⅓ cup	20.0
(Kellogg's):		
All-Bran	⅓ cup	21.0
Bran Buds	⅓ cup	22.0
Cracklin' Bran	⅓ cup	20.0
40% bran flakes	¾ cup	23.0
Raisin	¾ cup	28.0
(Nabisco) 100% bran	½ cup	21.0
(Post) 40% bran flakes	⅔ cup	22.6
(Post) raisin	½ cup	21.4
(Quaker) *Corn Bran*	⅔ cup	23.3
(Ralston Purina):		
Bran Chex	⅔ cup	23.0
Honey	⅞ cup	24.0
Raisin	¾ cup	30.0
(Shoprite) 40% bran flakes	⅝ cup	21.9
(Van Brode) 40% bran flakes	⅝ cup	21.9
BRANDY, FLAVORED		
(Mr. Boston):		
Apricot	1 fl. oz.	8.9
Blackberry	1 fl. oz.	8.6
Cherry	1 fl. oz.	7.4
Coffee	1 fl. oz.	10.6
Ginger	1 fl. oz.	3.5
Peach	1 fl. oz.	8.9
BRAN, MILLER'S (Elam's)	1 oz.	13.7

Food and Description	Measure or Quantity	Carbohydrates (grams)
BRAUNSCHWEIGER:		
(Oscar Mayer) chub	1-oz. serving	1.0
(Swift) 8-oz. chub	1-oz. serving	1.4
BRAZIL NUT:		
Shelled	4 nuts	1.9
Roasted (Fisher) salted	1-oz. serving	3.1
BREAD:		
American Granary (Arnold)	.9-oz. slice	12.5
Boston Brown	3" x ¾" slice	21.9
Bran'nola (Arnold)	1.2-oz. slice	15.5
Cinnamon raisin (Thomas')	.8-oz. slice	11.7
Cracked wheat (Pepperidge Farm)	1 slice	13.0
Crispbread, *Wasa:*		
Mora	1 slice	70.5
Rye:		
Golden	.4-oz. slice	7.8
Lite	.3-oz. slice	6.3
Sesame	.5-oz. slice	10.6
Sport	.4-oz. slice	9.1
Date nut roll (Dromedary)	1-oz. slice	13.0
Flatbread, *Ideal:*		
Bran	5-gram slice	4.1
Extra thin	.1-oz. slice	2.5
Whole grain	.2-oz. slice	4.0
French:		
(Pepperidge Farm)	2-oz. serving	27.0
(Wonder)	1-oz. slice	13.6
Hillbilly	1-oz. slice	12.5
Hollywood, dark	1-oz. slice	12.5
Honey bran (Pepperidge Farm)	1 slice	13.0
Honey, wheat berry (Arnold)	1.2-oz. slice	16.0
Italian (Pepperidge Farm)	2-oz. slice	28.0
Low sodium (Wonder)	1-oz. slice	13.5
Naturel (Arnold)	.9-oz. slice	12.0
Oatmeal (Pepperidge Farm)	1 slice	12.5
Profile (Wonder) dark	1-oz. slice	12.5
Protogen Protein (Thomas')	.7-oz. slice	8.5
Pumpernickel:		
(Arnold)	1-oz. slice	14.0
(Levy's)	1-oz. slice	14.0
(Pepperidge Farm):		
Regular	1 slice	15.0
Party	1 slice	3.0
Raisin:		
(Arnold) Tea	.9-oz. slice	13.0
(Pepperidge Farm) with cinnamon	1 slice	13.5
(Sun-Maid)	1-oz. slice	14.5

Food and Description	Measure or Quantity	Carbohydrates (grams)
Roman Meal	1-oz. slice	13.6
Rye:		
(Arnold) Jewish	1.1-oz. slice	14.0
(Levy's) real	1-oz. slice	12.0
(Pepperidge Farm) family	1 slice	15.0
(Wonder)	1-oz. slice	13.4
Sahara (Thomas'):		
Wheat	1-oz. piece	14.0
White	1-oz. piece	16.0
Sour Dough, *Di Carlo*	1-oz. slice	13.5
Wheat:		
Fresh Horizons	1-oz. slice	9.8
Fresh & Natural	1-oz. slice	13.6
Home Pride	1-oz. slice	13.1
(Pepperidge Farm)	1.2-oz. slice	17.5
(Wonder):		
Regular or cracked	1-oz. slice	13.6
100% whole wheat	1-oz. slice	11.9
Wheatberry, *Home Pride*	1-oz. slice	12.5
Wheat Germ (Pepperidge Farm)	1 slice	12.0
White:		
(Arnold) *Brick Oven*	.8-oz. slice	11.0
(Arnold) Melba thin	.5-oz. slice	7.0
Home Pride	1-oz. slice	13.1
(Levy's) no salt added	.9-oz. slice	14.0
(Pepperidge Farm):		
Large loaf	1 slice	13.0
Sandwich	1 slice	11.5
Sliced, 8-oz. loaf	.8-oz. slice	10.5
Sliced, 1-lb. loaf	.9-oz. slice	12.5
Sliced, very thin	1 slice	7.5
Toasting	1 slice	15.5
(Wonder) regular or buttermilk	1-oz. slice	13.6
Whole wheat:		
(Arnold) *Brick Oven*	.8-oz. slice	9.5
(Arnold) Melba thin	½-oz. slice	6.5
(Pepperidge Farm) thin slice	1 slice	12.0
(Thomas') 100%	.8-oz. slice	10.1
BREAD, CANNED, brown, plain or raisin (B&M)	½" slice	18.0
BREAD CRUMBS (Contadina) seasoned	½ cup	44.3
*BREAD DOUGH, frozen (Rich's):		
French	1⁄20 of loaf	11.0
Italian	1⁄20 of loaf	11.0
Raisin	1⁄20 of loaf	12.3
Wheat	.5-oz. slice	10.5
White	.8-oz. slice	9.4

Food and Description	Measure or Quantity	Carbohydrates (grams)
*BREAD MIX (Pillsbury):		
Applesauce spice, cranberry or nut	1/12 of loaf	28.0
Apricot nut or banana	1/12 of loaf	27.0
Blueberry nut	1/12 of loaf	26.0
Cherry nut	1/12 of loaf	30.0
Date	1/12 of loaf	32.0
BREAD PUDDING, with raisins	1/2 cup	37.6
BREAKFAST BAR (Carnation):		
Almond crunch, chocolate chip	1 piece	20.0
Chocolate crunch, peanut butter crunch	1 piece	22.0
BREAKFAST DRINK:		
(Ann Page)	2 tsps.	15.9
*(Pillsbury)	1 pouch	38.0
BREAKFAST SQUARES (General Mills) all flavors	1 bar	22.5
BREATH MINTS, dietetic (Featherweight)	1 piece	1.0
BRIGHT & EARLY	6 fl. oz.	21.6
BROCCOLI:		
Boiled, whole stalk	1 stalk	8.1
Boiled, 1/2" pieces	1/2 cup	3.5
Frozen:		
(Birds Eye):		
In cheese sauce	1/3 of pkg.	8.0
In Hollandaise sauce	1/3 of pkg.	2.9
(Green Giant):		
Spears in butter sauce	1/3 of pkg.	3.7
In cheese sauce, Bake 'n Serve	1/3 of pkg.	5.6
In cream sauce	1/2 cup	8.5
(McKenzie) chopped or spears	1/3 of pkg.	4.1
(Mrs. Paul's) in cheese sauce	1/3 of pkg.	18.6
(Seabrook Farms) chopped or spears	1/3 of pkg.	4.1
(Stouffer's) au gratin	1/3 of pkg.	6.9
BROTH & SEASONING:		
(George Washington)	1 packet	1.0
Maggi	1 T.	.1
BRUSSELS SPROUT:		
Boiled	3-4 sprouts	4.9
Frozen:		
(Birds Eye)	1/3 of pkg.	5.0
(Birds Eye) baby sprouts	1/3 of pkg.	5.8
(Green Giant):		
In butter sauce	1/3 of pkg.	5.0
Halves in cheese sauce	1/3 of pkg.	6.6
(Kounty Kist)	1/6 of pkg.	7.3
(Stouffer's) au gratin	1/3 of pkg.	16.0

Food and Description	Measure or Quantity	Carbohydrates (grams)
BUCKWHEAT, cracked (Pocono)	1 oz.	19.4
BUC*WHEATS, cereal (General Mills)	1 oz.	23.0
BULGUR, canned, seasoned	4-oz. serving	37.2
BURGER KING:		
Apple pie	3-oz. pie	32.0
Cheeseburger	1 burger	30.0
Cheeseburger, double meat	1 burger	32.0
Coca Cola	1 medium-size soda	31.0
French fries	1 regular order	25.0
Hamburger	1 burger	29.0
Onion rings	1 regular order	29.0
Shake:		
Chocolate	1 shake	57.0
Vanilla	1 shake	52.0
Whopper:		
Regular	1 burger	50.0
Regular, with cheese	1 burger	52.0
Double beef	1 burger	52.0
Double beef, with cheese	1 burger	54.0
Junior	1 burger	31.0
Junior, with cheese	1 burger	32.0
BURGUNDY WINE:		
(Gallo)	3 fl. oz.	1.2
(Great Western)	3 fl. oz.	2.3
(Italian Swiss Colony)	3 fl. oz.	.9
(Louis M. Martini)	3 fl. oz.	.2
(Paul Masson)	3 fl. oz.	2.2
(Taylor)	3 fl. oz.	3.3
BURGUNDY WINE, SPARKLING:		
(B&G)	3 fl. oz.	2.2
(Great Western)	3 fl. oz.	5.1
(Taylor)	3 fl. oz.	4.2
BURRITO:		
*Canned (Del Monte)	1 burrito	39.0
Frozen:		
(Hormel):		
Beef	1 burrito	28.4
Cheese	1 burrito	32.7
Hot chili	1 burrito	32.0
(Van de Kamp's) & guacamole sauce	½ of 12-oz. pkg.	40.0
BURRITO FILLING MIX, canned (Del Monte)	1 cup	39.0
BUTTER:		
Regular:		
(Breakstone)	1 T.	<.1
(Meadow Gold)	1 tsp.	0.

Food and Description	Measure or Quantity	Carbohydrates (grams)
Whipped (Breakstone)	1 T.	.1
BUTTER BRICKLE ICE CREAM		
BAR (Heath), chocolate coated	2½-fl.-oz. serving	18.0
BUTTERNUT, shelled	1 oz.	2.4
BUTTERSCOTCH MORSELS		
(Nestlé)	1 oz.	19.0

C

Food and Description	Measure or Quantity	Carbohydrates (grams)
CABBAGE:		
Fresh, white, chopped	½ cup	4.4
Canned (Greenwood) red, solids & liq.	½ cup	13.0
Frozen (Green Giant) stuffed	7-oz. serving	16.5
CABERNET SAUVIGON (Paul Masson)	3 fl. oz.	.2
CAFE COMFORT, 55 proof	1 fl. oz.	8.8
CAKE:		
Regular, non-frozen:		
Plain, home recipe, with butter, and boiled white icing	⅛ of 9" square	48.1
Plain, home recipe, with butter and chocolate icing	⅛ of 9" square	73.1
Angel food, home recipe	1/12 of 8" cake	24.1
Caramel, home recipe, with caramel icing	⅛ of 9" square	50.2
Chocolate, home recipe, with chocolate icing, 2-layer	1/12 of 9" cake	55.2
Crumb (Hostess)	1¼-oz. cake	21.7
Fruit:		
Home recipe, dark	1/30 of 8" loaf	9.0
Home recipe, light, made with butter	1/30 of 8" loaf	8.6
(Holland Honey Cake) unsalted	1/14 of cake	19.0
Pound, home recipe, traditional, made with butter	3½" x 3½" slice	14.1
Raisin Date Loaf (Holland Honey Cake) low sodium	1/14 of 13-oz. cake	19.0
Sponge, home recipe	1/12 of 10" cake	35.7
White, home recipe, made with butter, without icing, 2-layer	⅛ of 9" wide, 3" high cake	50.8
White, home recipe, made with butter, coconut icing, 2-layer	1/12 of 9" wide, 3¼" high cake	63.1

Food and Description	Measure or Quantity	Carbohydrates (grams)
Yellow, home recipe, made with butter, without icing, 2-layer	1/19 of cake	56.3
Frozen:		
Apple walnut (Sara Lee)	1/8 of 12½-oz. cake	21.6
Banana (Sara Lee)	1/8 of 13¾-oz. cake	26.9
Banana nut (Sara Lee) layer	1/8 of 20-oz. cake	26.5
Black forest (Sara Lee)	1/8 of 21-oz. cake	27.9
Carrot (Sara Lee)	1/8 of 12¼-oz. cake	18.9
Cheesecake:		
(Morton) *Great Little Desserts:*		
Cherry	6½-oz. cake	53.6
Cream	6½-oz. cake	46.2
Pineapple	6½-oz. cake	55.4
Strawberry	6½-oz. cake	57.2
(Rich's) Viennese	1/14 of 42-oz. cake	24.1
(Sara Lee):		
Blueberry, *For 2*	½ of 11.3-oz. cake	66.6
Cherry, *For 2*	½ of 11.3-oz. cake	69.3
Cream cheese:		
Blueberry	1/6 of 19-oz. cake	35.3
Cherry	1/6 of 19-oz. cake	35.2
French	1/8 of 23½-oz. cake	24.9
Large	1/6 of 17-oz. cake	25.9
Small	1/3 of 10-oz. cake	29.9
Strawberry	1/6 of 19-oz. cake	33.6
Strawberry, *For 2*	½ of 11.3-oz. cake	67.9
Strawberry French	1/8 of 26-oz. cake	27.5
Chocolate (Sara Lee)	1/8 of 13¼-oz. cake	28.1
Chocolate Bavarian (Sara Lee)	1/8 of 22½-oz. cake	22.6
Chocolate, German (Sara Lee)	1/8 of 12¼-oz. cake	19.3
Chocolate layer (Sara Lee) 'n cream	1/8 of 18-oz. cake	23.8
Coffee (Sara Lee):		
Almond	1/8 of 11¾-oz. cake	20.2
Almond ring	1/8 of 9½-oz. cake	16.8
Apple	1/8 of 15-oz. cake	24.1
Apple, *For 2*	½ of 9-oz. cake	58.1
Blueberry ring	1/8 of 9¾-oz. cake	17.6
Butter, *For 2*	½ of 6½-oz. cake	41.9
Maple crunch ring	1/8 of 9¾-oz. cake	17.3
Pecan, large	1/8 of 11¼-oz. cake	19.9
Pecan, small	¼ of 6½-oz. cake	22.1
Raspberry ring	1/8 of 9¾-oz. cake	18.5
Streusel, butter, large	1/8 of 11½-oz. cake	20.3
Streusel, cinnamon	1/8 of 10.9-oz. cake	19.0
Crumb (See ROLL or BUN)		
Orange (Sara Lee)	1/8 of 13¾-oz. cake	25.3

Food and Description	Measure or Quantity	Carbohydrates (grams)
Pound (Sara Lee):		
Regular	1/10 of 10¾-oz. cake	14.2
Banana nut	1/10 of 11-oz. cake	15.1
Chocolate	1/10 of 10¾-oz. cake	14.4
Chocolate swirl	1/10 of 11.8-oz. cake	16.0
Family size	1/15 of 16½-oz. cake	14.8
Home style	1/10 of 9½-oz. cake	13.1
Raisin	1/10 of 12.9-oz. cake	19.6
Strawberries & cream (Sara Lee) layer	1/8 of 20½-oz. cake	29.4
Strawberry shortcake (Sara Lee)	1/8 of 21-oz. cake	25.9
Torte (Sara Lee):		
Apple 'n cream	1/8 of 21-oz. cake	26.2
Fudge & nut	1/8 of 15¾-oz. cake	21.0
Walnut (Sara Lee) layer	1/8 of 18-oz. cake	22.8
CAKE or COOKIE ICING		
(Pillsbury) any flavor	1 T.	12.0
CAKE ICING:		
Butter pecan (Betty Crocker) *Creamy Deluxe*	½ of can	27.0
Caramel, home recipe	4-oz. serving	86.8
Cherry (Betty Crocker) *Creamy Deluxe*	1/12 of can	28.0
Chocolate:		
(Betty Crocker) *Creamy Deluxe:*		
Regular	1/12 of can	25.0
Fudge, dark dutch	1/12 of can	24.0
Milk	1/12 of can	26.0
Nut	1/12 of can	24.0
Sour cream	1/12 of can	25.0
(Pillsbury) *Frosting Supreme:*		
Fudge	1/12 of can	24.0
Milk	1/12 of can	25.0
Sour cream	1/12 of can	24.0
Cream cheese:		
(Betty Crocker) *Creamy Deluxe*	1/12 of can	27.0
(Pillsbury) *Frosting Supreme*	1/12 of can	27.0
Double dutch (Pillsbury) *Frosting Supreme*	1/12 of can	24.0
Lemon:		
(Betty Crocker) *Sunkist, Creamy Deluxe*	1/12 of can	28.0
(Pillsbury) ready-to-spread	1/12 of can	27.0
Orange (Betty Crocker) *Creamy Deluxe*	1/12 of can	28.0
Strawberry (Pillsbury) *Frosting Supreme*	1/12 of can	27.0

Food and Description	Measure or Quantity	Carbohydrates (grams)
Vanilla:		
(Betty Crocker) *Creamy Deluxe*	½₂ of can	28.0
(Pillsbury) *Frosting Supreme:*		
Regular	½₂ of can	27.0
Sour cream	½₂ of can	27.0
White:		
Home recipe, boiled	4-oz. serving	91.1
Home recipe, uncooked	4-oz. serving	92.5
(Betty Crocker) *Creamy Deluxe,*		
sour cream	½₂ of can	27.0
*CAKE ICING MIX:		
Regular:		
Banana (Betty Crocker)		
Chiquita, creamy	½₂ of pkg.	30.0
Butter Brickle (Betty Crocker)		
creamy	½₂ of pkg.	30.0
Butter pecan (Betty Crocker)		
creamy, deluxe	½₂ of pkg.	30.0
Caramel (Pillsbury) *Rich 'n Easy*	½₂ of pkg.	24.0
Cherry (Betty Crocker) creamy	½₂ of pkg.	30.0
Chocolate:		
(Betty Crocker) creamy:		
Fudge, regular or dark	½₂ of pkg.	30.0
Fudge, sour cream	½₂ of pkg.	30.0
Milk	½₂ of pkg.	30.0
(Pillsbury) *Rich 'n Easy:*		
Fudge	½₂ of pkg.	27.0
Milk	½₂ of pkg.	26.0
Coconut almond (Pillsbury)	½₂ of pkg.	17.0
Coconut pecan:		
(Betty Crocker) creamy	½₂ of pkg.	18.0
(Pillsbury)	½₂ of pkg.	20.0
Cream cheese & nut (Betty Crocker) creamy	½₂ of pkg.	23.0
Double dutch (Pillsbury) *Rich 'n Easy*	½₂ of pkg.	26.0
Lemon:		
(Betty Crocker) *Sunkist,* creamy	½₂ of pkg.	30.0
(Pillsbury) *Rich 'n Easy*	½₂ of pkg.	25.0
Strawberry (Pillsbury) *Rich 'n Easy*	½₂ of pkg.	25.0
Vanilla (Pillsbury) *Rich 'n Easy*	½₂ of pkg.	25.0
White:		
(Betty Crocker):		
Fluffy	½₂ of pkg.	16.0
Sour cream, creamy	½₂ of pkg.	31.0

23

Food and Description	Measure or Quantity	Carbohydrates (grams)
(Pillsbury) fluffy	1/12 of pkg.	17.0
Dietetic (Betty Crocker) *Lite:*		
Chocolate	1/12 of pkg.	18.0
Lemon and vanilla	1/12 of pkg.	19.0
CAKE MIX:		
Regular:		
Angel food:		
(Betty Crocker):		
Chocolate	1/12 of pkg.	32.0
One-step	1/12 of pkg.	32.0
Traditional	1/12 of pkg.	30.0
(Duncan Hines)	1/12 of pkg.	28.9
*(Pillsbury)	1/12 of cake	33.0
*Applesauce raisin (Betty Crocker) *Snackin' Cake*	1/9 of cake	33.0
*Applesauce spice (Pillsbury) *Pillsbury Plus*	1/12 of cake	34.0
*Banana:		
(Betty Crocker) *Supermoist*	1/12 of cake	36.0
(Pillsbury) *Pillsbury Plus*	1/12 of cake	36.0
*Banana walnut (Betty Crocker) *Snackin' Cake*	1/9 of cake	31.0
*Butter (Pillsbury):		
Pillsbury Plus	1/12 of cake	35.0
Streusel Swirl, rich	1/16 of cake	38.0
*Butter Brickle (Betty Crocker) layer, *Supermoist*	1/12 of cake	37.0
*Butter Pecan (Betty Crocker) *Supermoist*	1/12 of cake	35.0
*Butter yellow (Betty Crocker) *Supermoist*	1/12 of cake	36.0
*Carrot (Betty Crocker) *Supermoist*	1/12 of cake	34.0
*Carrot 'N Spice (Pillsbury) *Pillsbury Plus*	1/12 of cake	35.0
Cheesecake:		
*(Jell-O)	1/8 of 8" cake	33.0
*(Royal)	1/8 of cake	31.0
*Cherry chip (Betty Crocker) *Supermoist*	1/12 of cake	36.0
Chocolate:		
*(Betty Crocker):		
Pudding recipe	1/6 of cake	45.0
Snackin' Cake:		
Almond	1/9 of cake	31.0
Fudge chip	1/9 of pkg.	31.0
Stir 'N Frost:		
With chocolate frosting	1/6 of cake	38.0

24

Food and Description	Measure or Quantity	Carbohydrates (grams)
Fudge, with vanilla frosting	1/8 of cake	40.0
Supermoist:		
Fudge	1/12 of cake	35.0
German	1/12 of cake	36.0
Milk	1/12 of cake	35.0
Sour cream	1/12 of cake	36.0
*(Pillsbury):		
Bundt:		
Fudge nut crown	1/16 of cake	31.0
Fudge, triple	1/16 of cake	30.0
Fudge, tunnel of	1/16 of cake	37.0
Macaroon	1/16 of cake	35.0
Pillsbury Plus:		
Fudge, dark	1/12 of cake	35.0
Fudge, marble	1/12 of cake	36.0
German	1/12 of cake	36.0
Mint	1/12 of cake	33.0
Streusel Swirl, German	1/16 of cake	36.0
*Cinnamon (Pillsbury) Streusel Swirl	1/16 of cake	38.0
*Coconut pecan (Betty Crocker) Snackin' Cake	1/9 of cake	30.0
Coffee:		
*(Aunt Jemima)	1/8 of cake	29.0
*(Pillsbury):		
Apple cinnamon	1/8 of cake	40.0
Butter pecan	1/8 of cake	39.0
Cinnamon streusel	1/8 of cake	41.0
Sour cream	1/8 of cake	35.0
Devil's food:		
*(Betty Crocker) layer, Supermoist	1/12 of cake	35.0
(Duncan Hines) pudding recipe	1/12 of pkg.	34.8
*(Pillsbury):		
Pillsbury Plus	1/12 of cake	35.0
Streusel Swirl	1/16 of cake	36.0
Fudge (See CHOCOLATE)		
*Golden chocolate chip (Betty Crocker) Snackin' Cake	1/9 of cake	34.0
Lemon:		
*(Betty Crocker):		
Chiffon, Sunkist	1/12 of cake	35.0
Pudding	1/6 of cake	45.0
Stir 'N Frost, with lemon frosting	1/6 of cake	41.0
Supermoist	1/12 of cake	36.0

25

Food and Description	*Measure or Quantity*	*Carbohydrates (grams)*
(Duncan Hines) pudding recipe	1/12 of pkg.	36.1
*(Pillsbury):		
Bundt, tunnel of	1/16 of cake	43.0
Pillsbury Plus	1/12 of cake	36.0
Streusel Swirl	1/16 of cake	39.0
*Lemon blueberry (Pillsbury) *Bundt*	1/16 of cake	28.0
*Marble:		
(Betty Crocker) layer, *Supermoist*	1/12 of cake	40.0
(Pillsbury):		
Bundt, supreme	1/16 of cake	38.0
Streusel Swirl, fudge	1/16 of cake	38.0
*Orange (Betty Crocker) *Supermoist*	1/12 of cake	36.0
*Pound:		
(Betty Crocker) golden	1/12 of cake	27.0
(Dromedary)	3/4" slice	29.0
(Pillsbury) *Bundt*	1/16 of cake	33.0
*Spice (Betty Crocker):		
Snackin' Cake, raisin	1/9 of cake	33.0
Stir 'N Frost, with vanilla frosting	1/6 of cake	40.0
Supermoist	1/12 of cake	36.0
*Upside down (Betty Crocker) pineapple	1/9 of cake	43.0
White:		
*(Betty Crocker) *Stir 'N Frost*, with chocolate frosting	1/6 of cake	40.0
(Duncan Hines):		
Regular	1/12 of pkg.	34.8
Pudding recipe	1/12 of pkg.	36.5
*(Pillsbury) *Pillsbury Plus*	1/12 of cake	35.0
Yellow:		
*(Betty Crocker) *Supermoist*	1/12 of cake	37.0
(Duncan Hines):		
Regular	1/12 of pkg.	35.6
Pudding recipe	1/12 of pkg.	37.0
*(Pillsbury) *Pillsbury Plus*	1/12 of cake	36.0
*Dietetic:		
Chocolate:		
(Betty Crocker) *Light Style*, fudge	1/12 of cake	30.0
(Estee)	1/10 of cake	20.7
Devil's food (Betty Crocker) *Light Style*	1/12 of cake	29.0

Food and Description	Measure or Quantity	Carbohydrates (grams)
Lemon:		
(Betty Crocker) *Light Style*	1/12 of cake	29.0
(Estee)	1/10 of cake	19.1
Yellow (Betty Crocker) *Light Style*	1/12 of cake	29.0
White (Estee)	1/10 of cake	17.9
CAMPARI, 45 proof	1 fl. oz.	7.1
CANDY, REGULAR:		
Almond, chocolate covered (Hershey's) *Golden Almond*	1-oz. serving	12.4
Almond Cluster (Heath)	1 oz.	17.0
Almond, Jordan (Banner's)	1¼-oz. box	27.9
Baby Ruth	1.8-oz. piece	31.0
Breath Saver (Life Savers)	1 piece	1.7
Bridge mix (Nabisco)	1 piece	1.4
Bun Bars (Wayne)	1-oz. serving	17.0
Butter Brickle Bar (Heath)	1 oz.	17.0
Butterfinger	1.6-oz. bar	28.0
Butterscotch Skimmers (Nabisco)	1 piece	5.7
Candy corn (Brach's)	1 piece	1.8
Caramel:		
Caramel Flipper (Wayne)	1-oz. serving	19.0
Carmel Nip (Pearson)	1 piece	5.6
Caramel Pattie (Heath)	1-oz. serving	17.0
Cereal Raisin Bar (Heath)	2-oz. serving	37.0
Charleston Chew	1½-oz. bar	32.6
Cherry, chocolate-covered:		
(Nabisco)	1 piece	13.2
Welch's	1 piece	13.2
Welch's, milk	1 piece	13.1
Chocolate bar:		
Choco'Lite (Nestlé)	.27-oz. bar	4.9
Choco'Lite (Nestlé)	1-oz. serving	18.0
Crunch (Nestlé)	1 1/16-oz. bar	19.1
Crunch (Nestlé)	2½-oz. bar	45.0
Krunch (Heath)	1½-oz. serving	28.0
Milk:		
(Heath) crunch with toffee	2¼-oz. serving	42.0
(Heath) solid	2¼-oz. serving	41.0
(Hershey's)	1.2-oz. bar	19.4
(Hershey's)	4-oz. bar	64.7
(Nestlé)	.35-oz. miniature	5.6
(Nestlé)	1 1/16-oz. bar	18.0
Special Dark (Hershey's)	1.05-oz. bar	18.4
Special Dark (Hershey's)	4-oz. bar	70.2
Chocolate bar with almonds:		
(Heath)	2½-oz. serving	39.0
(Hershey's) milk	.35-oz. miniature	5.4

27

Food and Description	Measure or Quantity	Carbohydrates (grams)
(Hershey's) milk	1.15-oz. bar	17.6
(Hershey's) milk	4-oz. bar	61.4
(Nestlé)	1-oz. serving	17.0
(Nestlé)	5-oz. bar	85.0
Chocolate Parfait (Pearson)	1 piece	6.2
Chuckles	1-oz. serving	23.0
Circus Peanuts (Curtiss)	1 piece	6.0
Clark Bar	.7-oz. bar	14.2
Clark Bar	1.4-oz. bar	28.4
Clark Bar	1.65-oz. bar	33.4
Coconut bar, *Welch's*	1 piece	21.8
Coffee Nip (Pearson)	1 piece	5.6
Coffioca (Pearson)	1 piece	5.2
Crispy Bar (Clark)	1¼-oz. bar	24.2
Crispy Bar (Clark)	1.4-oz. bar	27.1
Crows (Mason)	1 piece	2.7
Dots (Mason)	1 piece	2.7
Dutch Treat Bar (Clark)	1 1/16-oz. bar	20.3
Dutch Treat Bar (Clark)	1.3-oz. bar	24.9
Frappe, *Welch's*	1 piece	23.5
Fruit Gems (Sunkist)	1 piece	8.2
Fruit roll (Sahadi):		
Any flavor but strawberry	1-oz. serving	20.0
Strawberry	1-oz. serving	22.0
Fudge (Nabisco) bar, *Home Style*	1 bar	13.9
Good & Fruity	1-oz. serving	26.3
Good & Plenty	1-oz. serving	24.8
Hollywood	1½-oz. bar	28.9
Jelly bean (Curtiss)	1 piece	3.0
Jelly rings, *Chuckles*	1 piece	9.0
Jujubes, *Chuckles*	1 piece	3.3
Ju Jus:		
Assorted	1 piece	2.0
Coins or raspberries	1 piece	4.0
Kisses (Hershey's)	1 piece	2.8
Kit Kat	.6-oz. miniature	9.4
Kit Kat	1⅛-oz. bar	21.0
Krackel Bar	.35-oz. miniature	5.9
Krackel Bar	1.2-oz. bar	20.3
Krackel Bar	4-oz. bar	67.7
Licorice:		
Licorice Nips (Pearson)	1 piece	5.6
(Switzer) bars, bites or stix:		
Black	1-oz. serving	22.1
Cherry or strawberry	1-oz. serving	23.2
Chocolate	1 oz. serving	22.7
Twist:		
Black (American Licorice Co.)	1 piece	6.4

Food and Description	Measure or Quantity	Carbohydrates (grams)
Black (Curtiss)	1 piece	6.0
Red (American Licorice Co.)	1 piece	7.3
Life Savers, drop	1 piece	2.4
Life Savers, mint	1 piece	1.7
Lollipops (Life Savers)	.9-oz. pop	24.0
Lollipops (Life Savers)	.6-oz. pop	16.7
Malted milk balls (Brach's)	1 piece	1.6
Marathon (M&M/Mars, Snackmaster)	.4-oz. bar	8.5
Mars Bar (M&M/Mars)	1½-oz. serving	25.6
Marshmallow (Campfire)	1-oz. serving	24.9
Mary Jane (Miller):		
Small size	¼ oz.	3.2
Large size	1½ oz.	19.5
Milk Duds (Clark)	.75-oz. box	17.8
Milk Duds (Clark)	1¼-oz. box	29.6
Milk Duds (Clark)	1.4-oz. box	33.2
Milk Shake (Hollywood)	1¼-oz. bar	26.8
Milky Way (M&M/Mars)	.8-oz. bar	16.3
Milky Way (M&M/Mars)	1.9-oz. bar	38.7
Mint or peppermint:		
After dinner (Richardson):		
Jelly center	1-oz. serving	26.0
Regular	1 oz. serving	27.0
Chocolate-covered (Richardson)	1 oz. serving	27.0
Cool Mints (Curtiss)	1 piece	5.0
Jamaica or *Liberty Mints* (Nabisco)	1 piece	5.8
Meltaway (Heath)	1 oz.	16.0
Mighty Mint (Life Savers)	1 piece	.4
Mint Parfait (Pearson)	1 piece	5.2
Junior mint pattie (Nabisco)	1 piece	2.0
Peppermint pattie (Nabisco)	1 piece	12.5
Thin (Nabisco)	1 piece	8.1
M & M's:		
Peanut	1½-oz. serving	25.0
Plain	1½-oz. serving	27.7
Mr. Goodbar (Hershey's)	.35-oz. miniature	4.9
Mr. Goodbar (Hershey's)	1½-oz. bar	20.8
Mr. Goodbar (Hershey's)	4-oz. bar	55.6
Munch peanut bar (M&M/Mars, Snackmaster)	1½-oz. bar	19.0
$100,000 Bar (Nestlé)	9/16-oz. bar	10.6
$100,000 Bar (Nestlé)	1¼-oz. bar	23.7
Orange slices:		
(Curtiss)	1 piece	14.4
(Nabisco) *Chuckles*	1 piece	7.2
Payday (Hollywood)	1⅓-oz. bar	22.3

Food and Description	Measure or Quantity	Carbohydrates (grams)
Peanut, chocolate-covered:		
(Curtiss)	1 piece	1.0
(Nabisco)	1 piece	1.6
Peanut, French burnt (Curtiss)	1 piece	1.0
Peanut brittle (Planters):		
Jumbo Peanut Block Bar	1-oz. serving	23.0
Jumbo Peanut Block Bar	.4-gram piece	12.0
Peanut butter cup:		
(Boyer)	1½-oz. pkg.	17.4
(Reese's)	.6-oz. cup	8.7
Poms Poms (Nabisco)	1 piece	2.3
Raisin, chocolate-covered:		
(Curtiss)	1-oz. serving	20.0
(Nabisco)	1 piece	.6
Raisinets (BB)	5¢ size	15.4
Reggie Bar	2-oz. bar	29.0
Rolo (Hershey's)	1 piece	4.1
Royals (M&M/Mars) mint chocolate	1½-oz. serving	27.9
Sesame Crunch (Sahadi)	¾-oz. bar	7.0
Snickers	1.8-oz. bar	30.2
Spearmint leaves:		
(Curtiss)	1 piece	8.0
(Nabisco) *Chuckles*	1 piece	6.6
Starburst (M&M/Mars)	1.9-oz. serving	45.3
Stars, chocolate (Nabisco)	1 piece	1.6
Sugar Babies (Nabisco)	1 piece	1.3
Sugar Daddy (Nabisco)		
Caramel sucker	1 piece	26.4
Nugget	1 piece	6.0
Sugar Mama (Nabisco)	1 piece	18.6
Sugar Wafer (F & F)	1¼-oz. pkg.	26.0
Summit, cookie bar (M&M/Mars)	¾-oz. serving	11.6
Taffy:		
Salt Water (Brach's)	1 piece	6.8
Turkish (Bonomo)	1-oz. bar	24.4
3 Musketeers	.8-oz. bar	17.2
3 Musketeers	2-oz. serving	43.9
Toffee (Kraft) all flavors	1 piece	5.2
Toffee Brickle (Heath)	1 oz.	17.0
Tootsie Roll:		
Chocolate	.23-oz. midgee	5.3
Chocolate	¹⁄₁₆-oz. bar	14.3
Chocolate	¾-oz. bar	17.2
Chocolate	1-oz. bar	22.9
Chocolate	1¾-oz. bar	40.0
Flavored	.6-oz. square	3.8
Pop, all flavors	.5-oz. pop	12.5

Food and Description	Measure or Quantity	Carbohydrates (grams)
Pop drop, all flavors	4.7-gram piece	4.2
Twix, cookie bar (M&M/Mars)	.85-oz. serving	15.6
Twix, peanut butter cookie bar (M&M/Mars)	.8-oz. serving	12.2
Twizzlers:		
Cherry, strawberry	1-oz. serving	22.0
Chocolate	1-oz. serving	21.0
Licorice	1-oz. serving	20.0
U-No Bar (Cardinet's)	⅞-oz. bar	21.3
Whatchamacallit (Hershey's)	1.15-oz. bar	18.7
World Series Bar	1-oz. serving	21.3
Zagnut Bar (Clark)	.7-oz. bar	14.6
Zagnut Bar (Clark)	1⅜-oz. bar	28.7
Zagnut Bar (Clark)	1⅝-oz. bar	33.9
CANDY, DIETETIC:		
Carob bar, *Joan's Natural:*		
Coconut	1 section of 3-oz. bar	2.4
Coconut	3-oz. bar	28.4
Fruit & nut	1 section of 3-oz. bar	2.6
Fruit & nut	3-oz. bar	31.2
Honey bran	1 section of 3-oz. bar	2.8
Honey bran	3-oz. bar	34.0
Peanut	1 section of 3-oz. bar	2.3
Peanut	3-oz. bar	27.4
Chocolate or chocolate flavored bar:		
(Estee):		
Bittersweet	1 section of 2½-oz. bar	2.7
Bittersweet	2½-oz. bar	32.0
Coconut	1 section of 2½-oz. bar	7.4
Coconut	2½-oz. bar	88.3
Crunch	1 section of 2-oz. bar	2.7
Crunch	2-oz. bar	32.2
Fruit & nut	1 section of 2½-oz. bar	2.6
Fruit & nut	2½-oz. bar	31.3
Milk	1 section of 2½-oz. bar	2.6
Milk	2½-oz. bar	31.0
Toasted bran	1 section of 2½-oz. bar	2.7
Toasted bran	2½-oz. bar	32.6
(Featherweight)	1 piece	4.0
Chocolate bar with almonds (Estee) milk	1 section of 2½-oz. bar	2.4

Food and Description	Measure or Quantity	Carbohydrates (grams)
Chocolate bar with almonds (Estee) milk	2½-oz. bar	29.2
Estee-ets (Estee) with peanuts	1 piece	.9
Gum drops (Estee) any flavor	1 piece	.7
Hard:		
(Estee) any flavor	1 piece	2.7
(Featherweight) assorted	1 piece	3.0
Mint:		
(Estee) *Esteemints*	1 piece	1.1
(Sunkist):		
Mini mint	1 piece	.2
Roll mint	1 piece	.9
Peanut butter cup (Estee)	1 piece	3.3
Raisin (Estee) chocolate covered	1 piece	.6
Rice crisp bar (Featherweight)	1 piece	4.5
T.V. Mix (Estee)	1 piece	.6
CANNELLONI FLORENTINE, frozen (Weight Watchers) one-compartment	13-oz. meal	52.0
CANTALOUPE, cubed	½ cup	6.1
CAPERS (Crosse & Blackwell)	1 tsp.	.3
CAP'N CRUNCH, cereal (Quaker):		
Regular or crunchberries	¾ cup	22.9
Peanut butter	¾ cup	20.9
CARAWAY SEED (French's)	1 tsp.	.8
CARDAMOM SEED (French's)	1 tsp.	1.3
CARNATION INSTANT BREAKFAST	1 pkg.	23.0
CARROT:		
Raw	5½" x 1" carrot	4.8
Boiled, slices	½ cup	5.4
Canned, regular pack:		
(Del Monte) drained	½ cup	6.8
(Libby's) solids & liq.	½ cup	4.6
(Stokely-Van Camp) solids & liq.	½ cup	5.0
Canned, dietetic pack:		
(Featherweight) sliced, solids & liq.	½ cup	6.0
(S&W) *Nutradiet,* sliced, solids & liq.	½ cup	7.0
Frozen:		
(Birds Eye) with brown sugar glaze	⅓ of pkg.	14.6
(Green Giant) nuggets in butter sauce	⅓ of pkg.	6.0
(McKenzie)	⅓ of pkg.	8.1
(Seabrook Farms)	⅓ of pkg.	8.1

Food and Description	Measure or Quantity	Carbohydrates (grams)
CARROT PUREE, dietetic		
(Featherweight)	1 cup	15.0
CASABA MELON	1-lb. melon	14.7
CASHEW NUT:		
(Fisher) dry or oil roasted	1-oz. serving	8.3
(Planters):		
Dry roasted	1-oz. serving	9.0
Oil roasted	1-oz. serving	8.0
CATAWBA WINE:		
(Great Western) pink, 12% alcohol	3 fl. oz.	11.3
(Taylor) 12% alcohol	3 fl. oz.	9.0
CATSUP:		
Regular:		
(Del Monte)	1 T.	5.5
(Smucker's)	1 T.	4.5
Dietetic or low calorie:		
(Featherweight)	1 T.	1.0
(Tillie Lewis) *Tasti Diet*	1 T.	2.0
CAULIFLOWER:		
Raw or boiled buds	½ cup	2.6
Frozen:		
(Birds Eye)	⅓ of pkg.	3.7
(Green Giant) in cheese sauce, *Bake 'n Serve*	⅓ of pkg.	5.6
(Mrs. Paul's) light batter & cheese	⅓ of pkg.	15.3
(Seabrook Farms)	⅓ of pkg.	4.5
(Stouffer's) au gratin	5-oz. serving	10.9
CAVIAR:		
Pressed	1-oz. serving	1.4
Whole eggs	1 T.	.5
CELERY:		
1 large outer stalk	8″ x 1½″ at root end	1.6
Diced or cut	½ cup	2.1
Salt (French's)	1 tsp.	Tr.
Seed (French's)	1 tsp.	1.1
***CELERY SOUP,** cream of:*		
(Campbell)	10-oz. serving	10.0
(Rokeach):		
Made with milk	10-oz. serving	19.0
Made with water	10-oz. serving	12.0
CERTS	1 piece	1.5
CHABLIS WINE:		
(Gallo)	3 fl. oz.	3.0
(Great Western)	3 fl. oz.	2.3
(Inglenook) Navelle	3 fl. oz.	.1
(Paul Masson) reg. or light	3 fl. oz.	2.7

Food and Description	Measure or Quantity	Carbohydrates (grams)
CHAMPAGNE:		
(Bollinger)	3 fl. oz.	3.6
(Gold Seal) pink, extra dry	3 fl. oz.	2.6
(Great Western):		
Regular	3 fl. oz.	2.4
Brut	3 fl. oz.	3.4
Extra dry	3 fl. oz.	4.3
Pink	3 fl. oz.	4.9
(Lejon)	3 fl. oz.	2.5
(Mumm's):		
Cordon Rouge, brut	3 fl. oz.	1.4
Extra dry	3 fl. oz.	5.6
(Taylor) dry	3 fl. oz.	3.9
CHARLOTTE RUSSE, homemade recipe	4-oz. piece	38.0
***CHEDDAR CHEESE SOUP**		
(Campbell)	11-oz. serving	14.0
CHEERIOS, cereal (General Mills):		
Regular	1¼ cups	20.0
Honey nut	¾ cup	23.0
CHEESE:		
American or cheddar:		
Cube	1″ cube	.4
Laughing Cow	1 oz.	Tr.
(Sargengo):		
Midget, regular or sharp	1 oz.	1.0
Shredded, non-dairy	1 oz.	1.0
Wispride, sharp	1 oz.	1.5
Blue:		
(Frigo)	1 oz.	1.0
Laughing Cow:		
Cube	⅛ oz.	.1
Wedge	¾ oz.	.5
(Sargento) cold pack or crumbled	1 oz.	1.0
Brick (Sargento)	1 oz.	1.0
Camembert (Sargento)	1 oz.	.1
Colby:		
(Pauly) low sodium	1 oz.	.6
(Sargento) shredded or sliced	1 oz.	1.0
Cottage:		
Unflavored:		
(Bison):		
Regular	1 oz.	1.0
Dietetic	1 oz.	1.0
(Dairylea)	1 oz.	1.0
(Friendship)	1 oz.	1.0

Food and Description	Measure or Quantity	Carbohydrates (grams)
Flavored (Friendship):		
With Dutch apple	1 oz.	2.5
With garden salad	1 oz.	1.0
With pineapple	1 oz.	3.8
Cream:		
Plain, unwhipped:		
(Frigo)	1 oz.	1.0
Philadelphia Brand (Kraft)	1 oz.	.9
Plain, whipped, *Temp-Tee*		
(Breakstone)	1 T.	.2
Edam:		
(House of Gold; Sargento)	1 oz.	1.0
Laughing Cow	1 oz.	Tr.
Farmers (*Dutch Garden Brand;*		
Friendship, regular or unsalted;		
Sargento; *Wispride*)	1 oz.	1.0
Feta (Sargento) Danish, cups	1 oz.	1.0
Gjetost (Sargento) Norwegian	1 oz.	13.0
Gouda:		
(Frigo)	1 oz.	1.0
Laughing Cow, natural	1 oz.	Tr.
(Sargento) baby, caraway or		
smoked	1 oz.	1.0
Wispride	1 oz.	<1.0
Gruyere, *Swiss Knight*	1-oz. wedge	<1.0
Havarti (Sargento) creamy and		
60% milk	1 oz.	.2
Hot pepper (Sargento) sliced	1 oz.	1.0
Jarlsberg (Sargento) Norwegian,		
sliced	1 oz.	1.0
Kettle Moraine (Sargento) sliced	1 oz.	1.0
Limburger (Sargento) natural	1 oz.	93
Monterey Jack:		
(Frigo)	1 oz.	1.0
(Sargento) midget, Longhorn,		
shredded or sliced	1 oz.	1.0
Mozzarella:		
(Fisher) part skim milk	1 oz.	1.0
(Frigo) part skim milk	1 oz.	1.0
(Sargento) bar or rounds,		
shredded, square or whole		
milk	1 oz.	1.0
Muenster (Sargento) red rind	1 oz.	1.0
Nibblin Curds (Sargento)	1 oz.	1.0
Parmesan:		
(Frigo):		
Grated	1 T.	Tr.
Whole	1 oz.	1.0

35

Food and Description	Measure or Quantity	Carbohydrates (grams)
(Sargento):		
Grated, non-dairy	1 T.	2.3
Wedge	1 oz.	1.0
Pizza (Sargento) shredded or sliced, non-dairy	1 oz.	1.0
Pot (Sargento) regular, French onion or garlic	1 oz.	1.0
Provolone (Frigo; Sargento)	1 oz.	1.0
Ricotta:		
(Frigo) moist, part skim milk	1 oz.	.9
(Sargento) part skim or whole milk	1 oz.	1.0
Romano:		
(Frigo):		
Grated	1 T.	Tr.
Wedge	1 oz.	1.0
(Sargento) wedge	1 oz.	1.0
Roquefort, natural	1 oz.	.6
Samsoe (Sargento) Danish	1 oz.	.2
Scamorze (Frigo)	1 oz.	.3
Stirred curd (Frigo)	1 oz.	1.0
String (Sargento)	1 oz.	1.0
Swiss:		
(Fisher) natural	1 oz.	0.
(Frigo) domestic	1 oz.	0.
(Sargento) sliced domestic or Finland	1 oz.	1.0
Taco (Sargento) shredded	1 oz.	1.0
Washed curd (Frigo)	1 oz.	1.0
CHEESE FONDUE, Swiss Knight	1 oz.	1.0
CHEESE FOOD:		
American or cheddar:		
(Weight Watchers) colored or white	1-oz. slice	1.0
Wispride, cheddar:		
Regular	1 oz.	2.0
& blue cheese	1 oz.	2.0
Hickory smoked	1 oz.	3.0
& port wine	1 oz.	<1.0
Sharp	1 oz.	2.0
Cheez 'N Crackers (Kraft)	1.1-oz. piece	9.3
Cheez-ola (Fisher)	1 oz.	.5
Cracker Snack (Sargento)	1 oz.	2.0
Loaf, Count Down (Fisher)	1 oz.	3.0
Mun-chee (Pauly)	1 oz.	2.0
Pimiento (Pauly)	.8-oz. slice	.8
Swiss (Pauly)	.8-oz. slice	1.6
CHEESE PUFF, frozen (Durkee)	1 piece	3.0

Food and Description	Measure or Quantity	Carbohydrates (grams)
CHEESE SPREAD:		
American or cheddar:		
(Fisher)	1 oz.	2.0
(Nabisco) *Snack Mate*	1 tsp.	.4
(Pauly)	.8 oz.	1.2
Wispride, sharp	1 oz.	2.0
Cheese 'n bacon (Nabisco) *Snack Mate*	1 tsp.	.4
Count Down (Fisher)	1 oz.	3.0
Imitation (Fisher) *Chef's Delight*	1 oz.	3.0
Pimiento:		
(Nabisco) *Snack Mate*	1 tsp.	1.8
(Price's)	1 oz.	2.0
Sharp (Pauly)	.8-oz.	.9
Swiss, process (Pauly)	.8-oz.	1.2
CHEESE STRAW, frozen (Durkee)	1 piece	1.0
CHELOIS WINE (Great Western)	3 fl. oz.	2.2
CHENIN BLANC WINE (Inglenook)	3 fl. oz.	1.3
CHERRY, sweet:		
Fresh, with stems	½ cup	10.2
Canned, regular pack (Stokely-Van Camp) solids & liq., pitted	½ cup	11.0
Canned, dietetic pack, solids & liq.:		
(Diet Delight) with pits, water pack	½ cup	16.9
(Featherweight):		
Dark, water pack	½ cup	13.0
Light, water pack	½ cup	11.0
CHERRY, CANDIED	1 oz.	24.6
CHERRY DRINK:		
Canned:		
(Ann Page)	1 cup	30.9
(Hi-C)	6 fl. oz.	23.0
(Lincoln) cherry berry	6 fl. oz.	23.9
*Mix (Hi-C)	6 fl. oz.	18.0
CHERRY HEERING (Hiram Walker)	1 fl. oz.	10.0
CHERRY JELLY:		
Sweetened (Smucker's)	1 T.	13.5
Dietetic:		
(Featherweight)	1 T.	4.0
(Featherweight) artificially sweetened	1 T.	1.0
Slenderella	1 T.	6.0
CHERRY LIQUEUR (DeKuyper)	1 fl. oz.	8.5
CHERRY PRESERVE or JAM:		
Sweetened (Smucker's)	1 T.	13.5

Food and Description	Measure or Quantity	Carbohydrates (grams)
Dietetic:		
(Dia-Mel)	1 tsp.	0.
(Featherweight) red	1 T.	4.0
(S&W) *Nutradiet*, red, tart	1 T.	3.0
CHERRY SPREAD, low sugar		
(Smucker's)	1 T.	6.0
CHESTNUT, fresh, in shell	¼ lb.	38.6
CHEWING GUM:		
Sweetened:		
Bazooka, bubble	1 slice	4.5
Beechies, Chicklets, tiny size	1 piece	1.6
Beech Nut; Beeman's; Big Red; Black Jack; Clove; Doublemint; Freedent; Fruit Punch; Juicy Fruit; peppermint or sour lemon (*Clark*); spearmint		
(*Wrigley's*); *Teaberry*	1 stick	2.3
Dentyne	1 piece	1.2
Dietetic:		
Bazooka, sugarless	1 piece	Tr.
Care*Free	1 piece	1.7
(Estee)	1 piece	1.3
(Featherweight)	1 piece	1.0
CHEX, cereal (Ralston Purina):		
Rice	1⅛ cups	25.0
Wheat	⅔ cup	23.0
Wheat & raisin	¾ cup	30.0
CHIANTI WINE:		
(Antinori) Classico, or vintage	3 fl. oz.	6.3
Brolio Classico	3 fl. oz.	.3
(Italian Swiss Colony)	3 fl. oz.	2.9
(Louis M. Martini)	3 fl. oz.	.2
CHICKARINA SOUP (Progresso)	1 cup	8.0
CHICKEN:		
Broiler, cooked, meat only	3 oz.	0.
Fryer, fried, meat & skin	3 oz.	2.7
Fryer, fried, meat only	3 oz.	1.0
Fryer, fried, a 2½-pound chicken (weighed with bone before cooking) will give you:		
Back	1 back	2.7
Breast	½ breast	1.1
Leg or drumstick	1 leg	.4
Neck	1 neck	1.9
Rib	1 rib	.8
Thigh	1 thigh	1.2
Wing	1 wing	.8
Fried skin	1 oz.	2.6

Food and Description	Measure or Quantity	Carbohydrates (grams)
Hen & cock:		
Stewed, meat & skin	3 oz.	0.
Stewed, dark meat only	3 oz.	0.
Stewed, light meat only	3 oz.	0.
Stewed, diced	½ cup	0.
Roaster, roasted, dark or light meat, without skin	3 oz.	0.
CHICKEN A LA KING:		
Home recipe	1 cup	12.3
Canned, (Swanson)	5¼-oz. serving	9.0
Frozen:		
(Banquet) *Cookin' Bag*	5-oz. pkg.	10.4
(Green Giant) *Toast Topper*	5-oz. pkg.	7.7
(Stouffer's) with rice	4¼-oz. serving	18.9
(Weight Watchers)	10-oz. bag	17.0
CHICKEN BOUILLON:		
(Croydon House)	1 tsp.	2.0
(Herb-Ox)	1 cube	.6
(Herb-Ox) instant	1 packet	1.9
(Maggi)	1 cube	1.0
MBT	1 packet	2.0
CHICKEN, CANNED, BONED:		
(Hormel) chunk	6¾-oz. serving	.8
(Swanson) chunk	2½-oz. serving	0.
CHICKEN, CREAMED, frozen		
(Stouffer's)	6½-oz. serving	5.9
CHICKEN CROQUETTE DINNER, frozen (Morton)	10¼-oz. dinner	46.5
CHICKEN DINNER or ENTREE:		
Canned (Swanson) & dumplings	7½-oz. serving	18.0
Frozen:		
(Banquet):		
& dumplings, *Buffet Supper*	2-lb. bag	128.2
& dumplings	12-oz. dinner	36.4
Man Pleaser	12-oz. dinner	89.2
(Green Giant):		
& biscuits	7-oz. serving	18.7
& biscuits, *Bake 'n Serve*	7-oz. entree	19.0
& noodles, boil-in-bag	9-oz. cooking bag	24.0
(Morton):		
Boneless:		
Regular	10-oz. dinner	22.8
King size	17-oz. dinner	53.1
Country Table:		
Regular	15-oz. dinner	94.8
Fried	12-oz. entree	27.3
& dumplings	11-oz. dinner	31.2
Fried	11-oz. dinner	50.0

Food and Description	Measure or Quantity	Carbohydrates (grams)
(Mrs. Paul's) pattie, breaded & fried with french fries	8½-oz. pkg.	51.3
(Stouffer's) cacciatore, with spaghetti	11¼-oz. meal	28.8
(Swanson):		
Hungry Man:		
Boneless	19-oz. dinner	74.0
Fried	15¾-oz. dinner	78.0
Fried	12-oz. entree	37.0
Fried, barbecue flavor	16½-oz. dinner	72.0
Fried, barbecue flavor	12-oz. entree	43.0
TV Brand:		
Fried	11½-oz. dinner	48.0
Fried, barbecue flavor	11¼-oz. dinner	47.0
Fried, crispy	10¾-oz. dinner	51.0
Fried, with whipped potatoes	7-oz. entree	25.0
Nibbles, with french fries	6-oz. entree	31.0
3-course	15-oz. dinner	65.0
In white wine sauce	8¼-oz. entree	10.0
(Weight Watchers):		
New Orleans style	11-oz. bag	19.1
Oriental style	12-oz. bag	18.0
Parmigiana, 2-compartment	7¾-oz. pkg.	11.0
Sliced, in celery sauce, 2-compartment	8½-oz. pkg.	13.9
Sliced, with gravy & stuffing, 3-compartment	14¾-oz. pkg.	42.1
Southern fried patty, 2-compartment	6¾-oz. pkg.	11.0
Sweet & sour	9½-oz. bag	27.0
CHICKEN FRICASSEE, home recipe	1 cup	7.7
CHICKEN, FRIED, frozen:		
(Banquet)	11-oz. pkg.	48.4
(Banquet)	2-lb. pkg.	117.3
(Morton)	2-lb. pkg.	32.7
(Morton) breast portion	22-oz. pkg.	31.2
(Swanson):		
Assorted pieces	3.2-oz. serving	10.0
Breast	3.2-oz. serving	8.0
Nibbles (wing)	3.2-oz. serving	12.0
Take-out style	4-oz. serving	8.0
Thighs & drumsticks	3.2-oz. serving	18.0
CHICKEN LIVER & ONION, frozen (Weight Watchers) 2-compartment	9¼-oz. meal	10.0
CHICKEN LIVER PUFF, frozen (Durkee)	½-oz. piece	3.0

Food and Description	Measure or Quantity	Carbohydrates (grams)
CHICKEN & NOODLES, frozen:		
(Banquet) *Buffet Supper*	1-lb. pkg.	79.1
(Green Giant)	9-oz. pkg.	21.5
(Stouffer's):		
Escalloped	5¾-oz. serving	15.8
Paprikash	10½-oz. serving	31.9
CHICKEN, PACKAGED (Louis Rich) breast, oven roasted	1 oz.	<1.0
CHICKEN PIE, frozen:		
(Banquet)	8-oz. pie	39.0
(Morton)	8-oz. pie	39.5
(Stouffer's)	10-oz. pie	39.8
(Swanson):		
Regular	8-oz. pie	42.0
Hungry Man	1-lb. pie	66.0
(Van de Kamp's)	7½-oz. pie	47.0
CHICKEN PUFF, frozen (Durkee)	½-oz. piece	3.0
CHICKEN SALAD (Carnation)	1½-oz. serving	2.6
CHICKEN SOUP, canned:		
Regular pack:		
*(Ann Page):		
Cream of	1 cup	9.3
& noodle	1 cup	8.7
& rice	1 cup	1.4
& stars	1 cup	7.4
(Campbell):		
Chunky:		
Regular	10¾-oz. can	22.0
Rice	9½-oz. can	15.0
Vegetable	9½-oz. can	19.0
*Condensed:		
Alphabet	10-oz. serving	12.0
Broth	10-oz. serving	4.0
Broth & noodles	10-oz. serving	10.0
Broth & rice	10-oz. serving	10.0
Broth & vegetables	10-oz. serving	7.0
Cream of	10-oz. serving	11.0
'N dumplings	10-oz. serving	12.0
Gumbo	10-oz. serving	10.0
Noodle	10-oz. serving	11.0
NoodleO's	10-oz. serving	11.0
Rice	10-oz. serving	9.0
Stars	10-oz. serving	9.0
Vegetable	10-oz. serving	10.0
Soup For One, semi-condensed:		
& noodle, golden	7¾-oz. can	14.0
vegetable, full flavored	7¾-oz. can	13.0

Food and Description	Measure or Quantity	Carbohydrates (grams)
(College Inn) broth	1 cup	0.
(Swanson) broth	7¼-oz. serving	1.0
Canned, dietetic pack:		
(Campbell):		
Chunky, low sodium	7½-oz. can	14.0
Noodle, low sodium	7¼-oz. can	8.0
*(Dia-Mel):		
Broth	8-oz. serving	1.0
& noodle	8-oz. serving	7.0
CHICKEN SOUP MIX:		
Carmel Kosher	6 fl. oz.	1.0
*(Lipton):		
Broth, *Cup-A-Broth*	6 fl. oz.	4.0
Cream of, *Cup-A-Soup*	1 pkg.	9.0
Giggle Noodle	1 cup	12.0
& noodle, with meat	1 cup	9.0
& rice	1 cup	8.0
Supreme, *Country Style*, *Cup-A-Soup*	6 fl. oz.	11.0
CHICKEN SPREAD, canned:		
(Swanson)	1-oz. serving	1.0
(Underwood)	1-oz. serving	1.1
CHICKEN STEW, canned:		
Regular pack:		
(Bounty)	7½-oz. serving	17.5
(Libby's) with dumplings	8-oz. serving	20.2
(Swanson)	7⅝-oz. serving	16.0
Dietetic or low calorie (Dia-Mel)	8-oz. can	19.0
CHICK 'N QUICK, frozen (Tyson):		
Breast pattie	¼ of 12-oz. pkg.	11.0
Breast fillet	¼ of 12-oz. pkg.	12.0
Chick 'N Cheddar	¼ of 12-oz. pkg.	12.0
Italian hoagie	¼ of 12-oz. pkg.	12.0
Turkey breast pattie	¼ of 12-oz. pkg.	11.0
CHICK PEAS or GARBANZOS, dry	1 cup	122.0
CHICORY, WITLOOF, cut	½ cup	.8
CHILI or CHILI CON CARNE:		
Canned regular pack:		
Beans only:		
(Blue Boy)	1 cup	46.0
(Van Camp) Mexican style	1 cup	43.0
With beans:		
(Hormel):		
Regular	7½-oz. serving	23.6
Short Orders, regular	7½-oz. can	24.0
Short Orders, hot	7½-oz can	23.0
(Libby's)	½ of 15-oz. can	32.2

42

Food and Description	Measure or Quantity	Carbohydrates (grams)
(Nalley's) mild or hot	8-oz. serving	27.3
(Swanson)	7¾-oz. serving	28.0
Without beans:		
(Hormel):		
Regular	7½-oz. serving	7.6
Short Orders	7½-oz. can	11.0
(Libby's)	½ of 15-oz. can	32.2
(Nalley's) *Big Chunk*	7½-oz. can	19.2
Canned, dietetic pack (Dia-Mel) with beans	8-oz. can	31.0
Frozen, with beans:		
(Stouffer's)	8¾-oz. pkg.	25.9
(Weight Watchers)	10-oz. pkg.	32.9
CHILI BEEF SOUP (Campbell):		
Chunky	11-oz. can	37.0
*Condensed	11-oz. serving	23.0
CHILI SAUCE, canned:		
Regular (Ortega) green	1 oz.	1.0
Dietetic (Featherweight)	1 T.	2.0
CHILI SEASONING MIX:		
*(Durkee)	1 cup	31.2
(French's) *Chili-O*	1 pkg.	30.0
CHIVES, raw	1 T.	.2
CHOCO-DILES (Hostess)	2.2-oz. piece	37.5
CHOCOLATE, BAKING:		
(Baker's):		
Bitter or unsweetened:		
Regular	1 oz.	8.6
Redi-Blend	1 oz.	8.0
Sweetened, *German's*	1 oz.	16.7
(Hershey's):		
Bitter or unsweetened	1 oz.	6.8
Sweetened:		
Dark, chips, regular or mini	1 oz.	17.8
Milk, chips	1 oz.	18.2
Semi-sweet, chips	1 oz.	17.3
(Nestlé):		
Bitter or unsweetened, *Choco-Bake*	1-oz. packet	12.0
Sweetened:		
Milk, morsels	1 oz.	17.0
Semi-sweet, morsels	1 oz.	18.0
CHOCOLATE, HOT, home recipe	1 cup	26.0
CHOCOLATE ICE CREAM:		
(Baskin-Robbins):		
Regular	2½ oz. (1 scoop)	20.4
Fudge	2½ oz. (1 scoop)	21.3
Good Humor, regular	4 fl. oz.	15.0

43

Food and Description	Measure or Quantity	Carbohydrates (grams)
(Meadow Gold)	¼ pt.	18.0
(Swift's)	½ cup	15.8
CHOCOLATE SYRUP (See SYRUP, Chocolate)		
CHOP SUEY, frozen:		
(Banquet) beef:		
Buffet Supper	2-lb. package	39.1
Cookin' Bag	7-oz. pkg.	9.5
(Stouffer's) beef, with rice	12-oz. serving	47.7
*CHOP SUEY SEASONING MIX (Durkee)	1¾ cups	21.0
CHOW CHOW:		
Sour	½ cup	4.9
Sweet	½ cup	33.1
CHOWDER:		
Canned, regular pack:		
Beef & vegetable (Hormel)	7½-oz. can	15.0
Chicken & corn (Hormel)	7½-oz. can	15.0
Clam:		
Manhattan style:		
(Campbell):		
Chunky	10¾-oz. can	23.0
*Condensed	10-oz. serving	15.0
(Crosse & Blackwell)	6½-oz. serving	9.0
New England style:		
*(Campbell):		
Condensed, made with milk	10-oz. serving	20.0
Condensed, made with water	10-oz. serving	13.0
Semi-condensed, *Soup For One*, made with milk	11-oz. serving	21.0
Semi-condensed, *Soup For One*, made with water	11-oz. serving	16.0
(Crosse & Blackwell)	6½-oz. serving	14.0
Ham 'N Potato (Hormel)	7½-oz. can	14.0
CHOW MEIN:		
Canned:		
(Chun King):		
Beef, *Divider Pak*	8-oz. serving	5.3
Chicken	8-oz. serving	6.7
Chicken, *Divider Pak*	10½-oz. serving	9.0
Pork, *Divider Pak*	12-oz. serving	7.0
Shrimp, *Divider Pak*	10½-oz. serving	8.0
(Hormel) pork, *Short Orders*	7½-oz. can	13.0

Food and Description	Measure or Quantity	Carbohydrates (grams)
(La Choy):		
Beef	1 cup	5.7
*Beef, bi-pack	1 cup	10.3
Chicken	½ of 1-lb. can	5.0
*Chicken, bi-pack	1 cup	9.3
Meatless	1 cup	5.9
*Mushroom, bi-pack	1 cup	10.7
Pepper Oriental	1 cup	10.2
*Pepper Oriental, bi-pack	1 cup	11.1
*Pork, bi-pack	1 cup	10.6
Shrimp	1 cup	5.7
*Shrimp, bi-pack	1 cup	9.7
Frozen:		
(Banquet) chicken, *Cookin' Bag*	7-oz. cooking bag	9.7
(Chun King):		
Chicken	11-oz. dinner	43.0
Shrimp	11-oz. dinner	43.0
(Green Giant) chicken	9-oz. entree	15.0
(La Choy):		
Beef, 5-compartment	11-oz. dinner	52.8
Beef entree	8-oz. serving	11.6
Chicken	11-oz. dinner	53.8
Chicken	8-oz. entree	9.1
Pepper Oriental	11-oz. dinner	54.6
Pepper Oriental	7½-oz. entree	11.5
Shrimp	11-oz. dinner	55.4
Shrimp	8-oz. entree	10.9
(Stouffer's) chicken	8-oz. serving	10.0
CINNAMON, ground (French's)	1 tsp.	1.4
CINNAMON LIFE, cereal (Quaker)	⅔ cup	19.7
CINNAMON SUGAR (French's)	1 tsp.	4.0
CITRUS COOLER DRINK, canned:		
(Ann Page)	1 cup	29.4
(Hi-C)	6 fl. oz.	23.0
CLAM:		
Raw, all kinds, meat only	1 cup (8 oz.)	13.4
Raw, soft, meat & liq.	1 lb. (weighed in shell)	5.3
Canned (Doxsee):		
Chopped or minced, solids & liq.	4 oz.	3.2
Chopped, meat only	4 oz.	2.1
Frozen (Mrs. Paul's):		
Deviled	3-oz. piece	14.4
Fried	2½-oz. serving	24.1
CLAMATO COCKTAIL, canned (Mott's)	6 fl. oz.	19.0
CLAM CHOWDER (See CHOWDER, Clam)		

Food and Description	Measure or Quantity	Carbohydrates (grams)
CLAM FRITTERS (See FRITTER, Clam)		
CLAM JUICE (Snow)	½ cup	1.2
CLAM SANDWICH, fried (Mrs. Paul's)	4½-oz. sandwich	54.3
CLARET WINE:		
(Gold Seal)	3 fl. oz.	.4
(Inglenook) Navelle	3 fl. oz.	.3
(Taylor) 12.5% alcohol	3 fl. oz.	2.4
CLORETS, gum or mint	1 piece	1.3
CLOVES (French's)	1 tsp.	1.2
COCOA:		
Dry unsweetened:		
(Hershey's)	1 T.	3.3
(Sultana)	1 T.	3.5
Mix:		
Regular:		
(Alba '66) instant, all flavors	1 envelope	11.0
(Carnation) all flavors	1-oz. pkg.	22.0
(Hershey's):		
Hot	1 oz.	21.0
Instant	3 T.	17.0
(Nestlé):		
Hot	1 oz.	23.0
With mini marshmallows	1 oz.	23.0
(Ovaltine) hot 'n Rich	1-oz. pkg.	22.0
Swiss Miss, regular or with mini marshmallows	6 fl. oz.	21.0
Dietetic:		
*(Featherweight)	6 fl. oz.	8.0
(Ovaltine) hot, reduced calorie	.45-oz. pkg.	8.0
Swiss Miss, instant, lite	3 T.	17.0
COCOA KRISPIES, cereal (Kellogg's)	¾ cup	25.0
COCOA PUFFS, cereal (General Mills)	1 cup	25.0
COCONUT:		
Fresh, meat only	2″ x 2″ x ½″ piece	4.2
Grated or shredded, loosely packed	½ cup	6.1
Dried:		
(Baker's):		
Angel Flake	¼ cup	7.9
Cookie	¼ cup	12.2
Premium shred	¼ cup	9.0
(Durkee) shredded	¼ cup	2.0
COCO WHEATS, cereal	1 T.	9.1
COD, broiled	3-oz. serving	0.

Food and Description	Measure or Quantity	Carbohydrates (grams)
COFFEE:		
Regular:		
*Max-Pax; Maxwell House; Maxwell House Electric Perk; Yuban; Yuban Electric Matic	6 fl. oz.	0.
*Mellow Roast	6 fl. oz.	2.0
Decaffeinated:		
*Brim; Sanka, regular or electric perk	6 fl. oz.	0.
*Brim, freeze-dried; Decaf, Nescafé, freeze-dried; Sanka, freeze-dried or instant	6 fl. oz.	1.0
*Freeze-Dried, Maxim; Sanka; Taster's Choice	6 fl. oz.	1.0
Instant:		
*Decaf; Nescafé; Sanka; Maxwell House; Sunrise	6 fl. oz.	1.0
*Mellow Roast	6 fl. oz.	2.0
*Mix (General Foods): Cafe Francais; Cafe Vienna; Irish Mocha Mint; Orange Cappuccino; Suisse Mocha	6 fl. oz.	7.0
COFFEE CAKE (See CAKE, Coffee)		
COFFEE SOUTHERN	1 fl. oz.	8.8
COLA SOFT DRINK (See SOFT DRINK, Cola)		
COLD DUCK WINE (Great Western) pink	3 fl. oz.	7.7
COLESLAW, made with mayonnaise-type salad dressing, solids & liq.	1 cup	8.5
COLLARDS:		
Leaves, cooked	½ cup	4.8
Canned (Sunshine) chopped, solids & liq.	½ cup	3.8
Frozen:		
(Birds Eye) chopped	⅓ of pkg.	4.0
(Southland) chopped	⅕ of 16-oz. pkg.	5.0
(Stouffer's) chopped	½ cup	4.3
COMPLETE CEREAL (Elam's)	1 oz.	17.5
CONCORD WINE:		
(Gold Seal)	3 fl. oz.	9.8
(Mogen David)	3 fl. oz.	16.0
CONSOMMÉ MADRILENE (Crosse & Blackwell):		
Clear	6½-oz. serving	4.0
Red	6½-oz. serving	0.

Food and Description	Measure or Quantity	Carbohydrates (grams)
COOKIE, REGULAR:		
Almond Windmill (Nabisco)	1 piece	7.0
Animal cracker:		
(Keebler):		
Regular	1 piece	1.9
100s, iced	1 piece	3.9
(Nabisco) Barnum's	1 piece	1.9
Apple Crisp (Nabisco)	1 piece	7.0
Assortment (Nabisco) Mayfair:		
Crown creme sandwich	1 piece	8.0
Fancy shortbread biscuit	1 piece	3.8
Filigree creme sandwich	1 piece	8.5
Mayfair creme sandwich	1 piece	9.0
Tea rose creme	1 piece	7.7
Tea time biscuit	1 piece	3.7
Biscos (Nabisco)	1 piece	6.0
Brown edge wafers (Nabisco)	1 piece	4.2
Brownie:		
(Frito-Lay) nut fudge	1.8-oz. piece	34.0
(Hostess)	1¼-oz. piece	24.1
(Sara Lee) frozen	⅛ of 13-oz. pkg.	26.1
Butter (Nabisco)	1 piece	3.5
Buttercup (Keebler)	1 piece	3.7
Butterscotch Chip (Nabisco) Bakers Bonus	1 piece	11.0
Caramel peanut log (Nabisco) Heyday	1 piece	13.0
Chocolate & chocolate-covered:		
(Keebler) fudge covered fudge stripes	1 piece	7.0
(Nabisco):		
Famous wafer	1 piece	4.6
Pinwheel, cake	1 piece	21.0
Snap	1 piece	2.8
Chocolate chip:		
(Keebler) Rich 'N Chips	1 piece	10.0
(Nabisco):		
Chips Ahoy!	1 piece	7.0
Chocolate	1 piece	7.3
Cookie Little	1 piece	1.0
Coconut:		
(Keebler) chocolate drop	1 piece	9.4
(Nabisco) bar, Baker's Bonus	1 piece	5.3
Devil's food cake (Nabisco)	1 piece	15.5
Double chips fudge (Nabisco)	1 piece	11.0
Fig bar:		
(Keebler)	1 piece	14.0

Food and Description	Measure or Quantity	Carbohydrates (grams)
(Nabisco):		
Fig Newtons	1 piece	11.0
Fig Wheats	1 piece	11.5
Gingersnaps (Nabisco) old fashioned	1 piece	5.5
Ladyfinger	3¼" x 1⅜" x 1⅛"	7.1
Lemon (Planters) creme	1 oz.	20.0
Macaroon, coconut (Nabisco)	1 piece	11.5
Marshmallow:		
(Nabisco):		
Mallomars	1 piece	8.5
Puffs, cocoa covered	1 piece	14.0
Sandwich	1 piece	5.7
Twirls, cakes	1 piece	20.0
(Planters) banana pie	1 oz.	22.0
Molasses (Nabisco) Pantry	1 piece	9.5
Nilla wafer (Nabisco)	1 piece	3.0
Oatmeal:		
(Keebler) old fashion	1 piece	12.0
(Nabisco):		
Bakers Bonus	1 piece	12.0
Cookie Little	1 piece	1.0
Peanut & peanut butter (Nabisco):		
Biscos	1 piece	5.7
Creme pattie	1 piece	3.8
Nutter Butter	1 piece	9.0
Peanut brittle (Nabisco)	1 piece	6.3
Pecan Sandies (Keebler)	1 piece	9.3
Raisin	1 oz.	22.9
Raisin (Nabisco) fruit biscuit	1 piece	12.0
Raisin Bar (Keebler) iced	1 piece	11.0
Sandwich:		
(Keebler):		
Chocolate fudge	1 piece	12.0
Elfwich	1 piece	8.1
Pitter Patter	1 piece	11.0
Vanilla creme	1 piece	8.5
(Nabisco):		
Brown edge	1 piece	10.0
Cameo	1 piece	10.5
Gaity, fudge	1 piece	7.0
Mystic Mint	1 piece	11.0
Oreo	1 piece	7.3
Oreo, double stuf	1 piece	9.0
Vanilla, Cookie Break	1 piece	7.3
Shortbread or shortcake (Nabisco):		
Cookie Little	1 piece	1.1
Lorna Doone	1 piece	5.0

Food and Description	Measure or Quantity	Carbohydrates (grams)
Melt-A-Way	1 piece	8.0
Pecan	1 piece	8.5
Striped	1 piece	6.3
Social Tea (Nabisco)	1 piece	3.5
Spiced wafers (Nabisco)	1 piece	5.8
Spiced Windmill (Keebler)	1 piece	9.2
Sugar cookie (Nabisco) rings		
Bakers Bonus	1 piece	10.5
Sugar wafer:		
(Dutch Treat)	1 piece	6.3
(Dutch Twin)	1 piece	6.2
(Keebler) Krisp Kreem	1 piece	4.2
(Nabisco) Biscos	1 piece	2.6
Vanilla creme (Planters)	1 oz.	20.0
Vanilla wafer (Keebler)	1 piece	2.6
Waffle creme (Dutch Twin)	1 piece	5.7
COOKIE, DIETETIC:		
Chocolate chip:		
(Estee)	1 piece	3.4
(Featherweight)	1 piece	4.0
Chocolate crescent		
(Featherweight)	1 piece	4.0
Coconut (Estee)	1 piece	2.7
Fudge (Estee)	1 piece	3.3
Lemon:		
(Estee) thin	1 piece	3.1
(Featherweight)	1 piece	4.0
Oatmeal raisin (Estee)	1 piece	3.3
Sandwich:		
(Estee):		
Duplex	1 piece	5.6
Lemon	1 piece	5.6
(Featherweight)	1 piece	6.0
Vanilla:		
(Estee) thin	1 piece	3.1
(Featherweight)	1 piece	4.0
Wafer:		
(Estee):		
Chocolate covered	1 piece	13.1
Chocolate-strawberry snack	1 piece	10.0
Creme, assorted	1 piece	4.2
Creme, chocolate	1 piece	2.8
Creme, vanilla	1 piece	2.8
Vanilla, snack, sugar-free	1 piece	10.1
Wheat germ	1 piece	1.3
(Featherweight) chocolate, peanut butter or vanilla creme	1 piece	4.0

Food and Description	Measure or Quantity	Carbohydrates (grams)
COOKIE CRISP, cereal (Ralston Purina)	1 cup	25.0
*COOKIE DOUGH:		
Refrigerated (Pillsbury):		
Brownie, fudge	1 brownie	39.0
Chocolate chip	1 piece	7.3
Oatmeal	1 piece	7.3
Peanut Butter	1 piece	6.3
Sugar	1 piece	7.7
Frozen (Rich's):		
Chocolate chip	1 piece	20.3
Sugar	1 piece	17.4
COOKIE MIX:		
Regular:		
Brownie:		
*(Betty Crocker):		
Chocolate chip butterscotch	¹⁄₁₆ of pkg.	21.0
Fudge	¹⁄₁₆ of pkg.	22.0
Fudge, family size	¹⁄₂₄ of pkg.	21.0
Fudge supreme	¹⁄₁₆ of pkg.	21.0
German chocolate	¹⁄₁₆ of pkg.	26.0
Walnut	¹⁄₁₆ of pkg.	22.0
Walnut, family size	¹⁄₂₄ of pkg.	19.0
(Duncan Hines)	¹⁄₂₄ of pkg.	19.4
*(Nestlé)	¹⁄₂₄ of pkg.	22.0
*(Pillsbury):		
Fudge	¹⁄₃₆ of pkg.	10.0
Fudge, family size	¹⁄₄₈ of pkg.	11.0
Walnut	¹⁄₃₆ of pkg.	10.0
Walnut, family size	¹⁄₄₈ of pkg.	11.5
Chocolate:		
*(Betty Crocker) *Big Batch*, double	1 piece	8.5
(Duncan Hines) double	¹⁄₃₆ of pkg.	9.2
Chocolate chip:		
*(Betty Crocker) *Big Batch*	1 piece	8.0
(Duncan Hines)	¹⁄₃₆ of pkg.	9.1
*(Nestlé)	1 piece	7.5
*(Quaker)	1 piece	8.5
*Date bar (Betty Crocker)	¹⁄₃₂ of pkg.	9.0
*Macaroon, coconut (Betty Crocker)	¹⁄₂₄ of pkg.	10.0
Oatmeal:		
*(Betty Crocker) *Big Batch*	1 piece	8.5
(Duncan Hines) raisin	¹⁄₃₆ of pkg.	9.1
*(Nestlé) raisin	1 piece	9.0
*(Quaker)	1 piece	9.3

Food and Description	Measure or Quantity	Carbohydrates (grams)
Peanut butter:		
*(Betty Crocker) *Big Batch*	1 piece	7.0
*(Betty Crocker) *Big Batch*, with flavored chips	1 piece	8.0
(Duncan Hines)	1/36 of pkg.	7.5
*(Nestlé)	1 piece	7.5
*(Quaker)	1 piece	8.0
Sugar:		
*(Betty Crocker) *Big Batch*	1 piece	9.0
(Duncan Hines) golden	1/36 of pkg.	8.4
*(Nestlé)	1 piece	8.5
*Vienna dream bar (Betty Crocker)	1/24 of pkg.	10.0
*Dietetic (Dia-Mel)	2″ cookie	7.0
COOKING SPRAY, *Mazola No Stick*	2-second spray	0.
CORIANDER, seed (French's)	1 tsp.	.8
CORN:		
Fresh, on the cob, boiled	5″ x 1¾″ ear	16.2
Canned, regular pack:		
(Del Monte):		
Cream style, golden, wet pack	½ cup	19.2
Whole kernel, drained	½ cup	21.3
Whole kernel, vacuum pack	½ cup	21.6
(Festal):		
Cream style, white, wet pack	½ cup	21.3
Whole kernel, white, drained	½ cup	21.4
(Green Giant):		
Cream style	4¼-oz. serving	22.3
Whole kernel, solids & liq.	4¼-oz. serving	15.8
Whole kernel, *Mexicorn*, solids & liq.	4-oz. serving	20.3
Whole kernel, *Niblets*, vacuum pack	4-oz. serving	19.5
(Le Sueur) solids & liq.	4¼-oz. serving	17.3
(Libby's):		
Cream style	½ cup	21.2
Whole kernel, solids & liq.	½ cup	18.8
(Stokely-Van Camp):		
Cream style	½ cup	23.5
Whole kernel, solids & liq.	½ cup	17.6
Canned, dietetic pack:		
(Blue Boy) cream style	4-oz. serving	22.0
(Diet Delight) solids & liq.	½ cup	15.0
(Featherweight) whole kernel, solids & liq.	½ cup	16.0
(S&W) *Nutradiet*, cream style	½ cup	21.0
(S&W) *Nutradiet*, whole kernel, solids & liq.	½ cup	15.0

Food and Description	Measure or Quantity	Carbohydrates (grams)
Frozen:		
(Birds Eye):		
On the cob	4.9-oz. ear	28.0
On the cob, *Little Ears*	1 ear	16.0
Whole kernel	⅓ of pkg.	18.0
(Green Giant):		
On the cob	5½″ ear	32.7
On the cob, *Nibbler*	3″ ear	18.0
Whole kernel, golden	4-oz. serving	20.5
Whole kernel, golden, in butter sauce, *Mexicorn* or *Niblets*	⅓ of pkg.	14.2
Whole kernel, white, in butter sauce	⅓ of pkg.	15.2
(McKenzie) whole kernel	⅓ of pkg.	19.9
(Ore-Ida):		
On the cob	1 ear	27.0
Whole kernel	3.2-oz. serving	21.3
(Seabrook Farms):		
On the cob	5″ ear	30.0
Whole kernel	⅓ of pkg.	19.9
CORNBREAD:		
Home recipe:		
Corn pone	4-oz. serving	41.1
Spoon bread	4-oz. serving	19.2
*Mix:		
(Aunt Jemima)	⅙ of pkg.	34.0
(Dromedary)	2″ x 2″ piece	19.0
(Pillsbury) *Ballard*	1/16 of recipe	26.0
CORN CHEX, cereal (Ralston Purina)	1 cup	25.0
CORN DOG, frozen:		
(Hormel)	1 wiener	22.0
(Hormel) *Tater Dogs*	1 wiener	15.0
(Oscar Mayer)	1 piece	27.9
CORNED BEEF:		
Cooked, boneless, medium fat	4-oz. serving	0.
Canned:		
Dinty Moore	3-oz. serving	0.
(Libby's)	3½-oz. serving	1.9
Packaged:		
(Eckrich) sliced	1-oz. slice	.9
(Oscar Mayer) jellied loaf	1-oz. slice	0.
(Vienna):		
Brisket	1-oz. serving	0.
Flats	1-oz. serving	.1
CORNED BEEF HASH, canned:		
(Libby's)	1 cup	31.1

Food and Description	Measure or Quantity	Carbohydrates (grams)
Mary Kitchen	7½-oz. serving	21.1
Mary Kitchen, Short Orders	7½-oz. can	16.0
(Nalley's)	4-oz. serving	10.2
CORNED BEEF HASH DINNER, frozen (Banquet)	10-oz. dinner	42.6
CORNED BEEF SPREAD (Underwood)	1-oz. serving	Tr.
CORN FLAKE CRUMBS (Kellogg's)	¼ cup	25.0
CORN FLAKES, cereal:		
(General Mills) Country	1 cup	25.0
(Kellogg's):		
Regular	1 cup	24.0
Honey & nut	¾ cup	24.0
Sugar frosted	¾ cup	26.0
King Kullen:		
Regular	1 cup	24.3
Sugar toasted	¾ cup	25.3
(Post) Post Toasties	1¼ cups	24.4
(Ralston Purina):		
Regular	1 cup	25.0
Sugar frosted	¾ cup	26.0
(Van Brode):		
Regular	1 oz.	24.4
Low sodium	1 oz.	25.0
Sugar toasted	1 oz.	25.3
CORN FRITTER (See FRITTER, Corn)		
CORN MEAL:		
Bolted (Aunt Jemima/Quaker)	3 T.	21.2
Degermed	¼ cup	27.5
Mix:		
Bolted (Aunt Jemima)	1 cup	80.4
Degermed (Aunt Jemima)	1 cup	84.0
CORNNUTS	1-oz. serving	21.0
CORN STARCH (Argo; Kingsford's; Duryea)	1 tsp.	2.4
CORN SYRUP (See SYRUP, Corn)		
CORN TOTAL, cereal (General Mills)	1 cup	24.0
COUGH DROP:		
(Beech-Nut)	1 drop	2.4
(Luden's)	1 drop	2.1
(Pine Bros.)	1 drop	2.0
(Smith Brothers)	1 drop	2.1
Dietetic (Estee)	1 drop	3.1
COUNT CHOCULA, cereal (General Mills)	1 cup	24.0

Food and Description	Measure or Quantity	Carbohydrates (grams)
COUNTRY CRISP, cereal (Post)	¾ cup	24.4
CRAB:		
Fresh, steamed:		
Whole	½ lb.	.6
Meat only	4-oz. serving	.6
Canned, king crab (Icy Point; Pillar Rock)	3¾-oz. serving	1.1
Frozen (Wakefield's Alaska King)	4-oz. serving	.6
CRAB APPLE	¼ lb.	18.5
CRAB APPLE JELLY (Smucker's)	1 T.	13.5
CRAB, DEVILED, frozen, breaded & fried (Mrs. Paul's) regular	3-oz. serving	17.0
CRAB IMPERIAL, home recipe	1 cup	8.6
CRAB SOUP (Crosse & Blackwell)	½ of 13-oz. can	8.0
CRACKED WHEAT CEREAL (Elam's)	1 oz.	20.2
CRACKERS, PUFFS & CHIPS:		
American Harvest (Nabisco)	1 piece	2.0
Arrowroot biscuit (Nabisco)	1 piece	3.5
Bacon 'n Dip (Nabisco)	1 piece	.9
Bacon-flavored thins (Nabisco)	1 piece	1.3
Bacon Nips	1 oz.	15.6
Bacon Toast (Keebler)	1 piece	2.0
Biscos (Nabisco)	1 piece	2.6
Bugles (General Mills)	1 oz.	18.0
Cheese flavored:		
Bops (Nalley's)	1 oz.	13.6
Cheddar Bitz (Frito-Lay)	1 oz.	18.9
Cheddar triangles (Nabisco)	1 piece	.9
Cheese balls (Planters)	1 oz.	4.3
Cheese curls (Planters)	1 oz.	4.3
Cheese 'n Crunch (Nabisco)	1 oz.	14.0
Cheese filled (Frito-Lay)	1½ oz.	25.3
Cheese Pixies (Wise) baked or fried	1 oz.	15.6
Chee•Tos, crunchy or puffed	1 oz.	15.0
Cheez Balls (Planters)	1 oz.	15.0
Cheez Curls (Planters)	1 oz.	15.0
Country Cheddar 'n Sesame (Nabisco)	1 piece	1.0
Nacho cheese cracker (Keebler)	1 piece	1.6
Sandwich (Planters)	1 piece	3.0
Swiss cheese (Nabisco)	1 piece	1.1
Tid-Bit (Nabisco)	1 oz.	.5
Twists (Bachman) baked	1 oz.	17.0
Twists (Nalley's)	1 oz.	9.1
Chicken in a Biskit (Nabisco)	1 piece	1.1

55

Food and Description	Measure or Quantity	Carbohydrates (grams)
Chip O' Cheddar, Flavor Kist (Schulze and Burch)	1 oz.	17.0
Chippers (Nabisco)	1 piece	.7
Chipsters (Nabisco)	1 piece	.3
Club cracker (Keebler)	1 piece	2.1
Corn chips:		
(Bachman) regular or BBQ	1 oz.	15.0
Fritos	1 oz.	16.0
Fritos, barbecue flavor	1 oz.	15.5
Korkers (Nabisco)	1 piece	.8
(Old London)	1 oz.	16.7
(Planters)	1 oz.	15.0
Corn Nuggets (Frito-Lay)	1 oz.	21.2
Corn Nuts (Nalley's)	1 oz.	10.4
Corn & Sesame Chips (Nabisco)	1 piece	.9
Creme Wafer Stick (Nabisco)	1 piece	6.3
Crown Pilot (Nabisco)	1 piece	13.0
Diggers (Nabisco)	1 piece	.5
Dixies (Nabisco)	1 piece	.9
Doo Dads (Nabisco)	1 piece	.3
Escort (Nabisco)	1 piece	2.7
Flings (Nabisco)	1 piece	.8
French onion cracker (Nabisco)	1 piece	1.5
Goldfish (Pepperidge Farm):		
Thins	1 piece	2.2
Tiny:		
All flavors but pretzel	¼-oz. serving	4.0
Pretzel	¼-oz. serving	5.0
Graham:		
Cinnamon Treat (Nabisco)	1 piece	5.0
Flavor Kist (Schulze and Burch) sugar-honey coated	1 double piece	10.0
Honey Maid (Nabisco)	1 piece	5.5
(Nabisco)	1 piece	5.3
Graham, chocolate or cocoa-covered:		
Fancy Dip (Nabisco)	1 piece	8.5
(Keebler)	1 piece	5.6
Lil' Loaf (Nabisco)	1 piece	1.8
Marzo (See MATZO)		
Melba toast (See MELBA TOAST)		
Milk Lunch Biscuit (Keebler)	1 piece	4.5
Mucho Macho Nacho, Flavor Kist (Schulze and Burch)	1 oz.	18.0
Onion Toast (Keebler)	1 piece	2.1
Oyster:		
(Keebler) Zesta	1 piece	.3
(Nabisco) Oysterettes	1 piece	.6

56

Food and Description	Measure or Quantity	Carbohydrates (grams)
Ritz (Nabisco)	1 piece	2.0
Roman Meal Wafer, boxed	1 piece	1.3
Royal Lunch (Nabisco)	1 piece	8.0
Rusk, *Holland* (Nabisco)	1 piece	7.5
Rye Toast (Keebler)	1 piece	2.1
Ry-Krisp, natural	1 triple cracker	5.0
Rye wafer (Nabisco)	1 piece	4.5
Saltine:		
Flavor Kist (Schulze and Burch)	1 piece	2.0
Hi-Ho (Sunshine)	1 piece	2.1
Premium (Nabisco)	1 piece	2.0
Zesta (Keebler)	1 piece	2.1
Sea Toast (Keebler)	1 piece	10.0
Sesame:		
Flavor Kist (Schulze and Burch) sesame wheat snacks	1 oz.	18.0
Butter flavored (Nabisco)	1 piece	1.9
Sesame Wheats! (Nabisco)	1 piece	1.8
Sticks (Keebler)	1 piece	.8
Teeko (Nabisco)	1 piece	3.0
Toast (Keebler)	1 piece	2.0
Shindigs (Keebler)	1 piece	.9
Skittle Chips (Nabisco)	1 piece	1.8
Snack sticks (Pepperidge Farm):		
Lightly salted	1 oz.	18.0
Pumpernickel	1 oz.	17.0
Sesame	1 oz.	16.0
Wheat	1 oz.	17.0
Soda (Nabisco) *Gitana*	1 piece	2.5
Table Water Cracker (Carr's) small	1 piece	2.6
Tater Puffs (Nabisco)	1 piece	.8
Tortilla chips:		
(Bachman) nacho or taco flavor	1 oz.	17.0
Buenos (Nabisco) nacho or taco flavor	1 piece	1.2
Doritas, nacho or taco flavor (Nabisco) regular and nacho flavor	1 oz.	18.0
	1 piece	1.3
(Planters) nacho or taco flavor	1 oz.	14.0
Tostitos	1 oz.	17.0
Town House Cracker (Keebler)	1 piece	1.8
Triscuit (Nabisco)	1 piece	3.0
Twigs (Nabisco)	1 stick	1.6
Uneeda Biscuit (Nabisco)	1 piece	3.7
Vegetable thins (Nabisco)	1 piece	1.3
Waldorf (Keebler)	1 piece	2.3
Waverly Wafer (Nabisco)	1 piece	2.6

Food and Description	Measure or Quantity	Carbohydrates (grams)
Wheat chips (Nabisco)	1 piece	.5
Wheat crisps (Keebler)	1 piece	1.7
Wheatmeal Biscuit (Carr's) small	1 piece	5.9
Wheat snacks, *Flavor Kist* (Schulze and Burch):		
Natural	1 oz.	16.0
Rye	1 oz.	17.0
Wild onion	1 oz.	18.0
Wheatsworth (Nabisco)	1 piece	1.8
Wheat Thins (Nabisco)	1 piece	1.2
Wheat Toast (Keebler)	1 piece	2.0
CRACKER CRUMBS, graham (Nabisco)	⅛ of 9″ pie shell	12.0
CRACKER MEAL (Nabisco)	½ cup	47.4
CRANAPPLE JUICE (Ocean Spray): canned:		
Regular	6 fl. oz.	32.1
Low calorie	6 fl. oz.	7.4
CRANBERRY, fresh (Ocean Spray)	½ cup	23.9
*CRANBERRY-APPLE JUICE, frozen (Welch's)	6 fl. oz.	30.0
*CRANBERRY-GRAPE JUICE, frozen (Welch's)	6 fl. oz.	27.0
CRANBERRY JUICE COCKTAIL: Canned (Ocean Spray):		
Regular	6 fl. oz.	26.4
Dietetic	6 fl. oz.	8.3
*Frozen (Welch's)	6 fl. oz.	26.0
CRANBERRY-ORANGE JUICE DRINK, canned (Ocean Spray)	6 fl. oz.	24.6
CRANBERRY-ORANGE RELISH (Ocean Spray)	1 T.	8.2
CRANBERRY-RASPBERRY SAUCE (Ocean Spray) jellied	2-oz. serving	20.8
CRANBERRY SAUCE:		
Home recipe	4 oz.	51.6
Canned (Ocean Spray):		
Jellied	2-oz. serving	21.7
Whole berry	2-oz. serving	22.0
CRANGRAPE, canned (Ocean Spray)	6 fl. oz.	26.2
*CRANORANGE, frozen (Ocean Spray)	6 fl. oz.	26.2
CRANPRUNE JUICE, canned (Ocean Spray)	6 fl. oz.	28.8
CRAZY COW, cereal (General Mills)	1 cup	24.0

Food and Description	Measure or Quantity	Carbohydrates (grams)
CREAM:		
Half & Half (Dairylea)	1 fl. oz.	1.0
Light, table or coffee (Sealtest)	1 T.	.6
Light whipping, 30% fat (Sealtest)	1 T.	1.0
Heavy whipping (Dairylea)	1 fl. oz.	1.0
Sour (Dairylea)	1 fl. oz.	1.0
Sour, imitation (Pet)	1 T.	1.0
Substitute (See CREAM SUBSTITUTE)		
CREAM PUFFS:		
Home recipe, custard filling	3½" x 2" piece	26.7
Frozen (Rich's) chocolate	1⅓-oz. piece	16.9
CREAM OF RICE, cereal	4-oz. serving	17.9
CREAMSICLE (Popsicle Industries)	2½-fl.-oz. piece	13.0
CREAM SUBSTITUTE:		
Coffee Rich	½ oz.	2.1
Coffee Twin	½ fl. oz.	1.0
Dairy Light (Alba)	2.8-oz. envelope	1.0
N-Rich	1½ tsp.	1.7
Perx	1 tsp.	.6
(Pet)	1 tsp.	1.0
Poly Perx	½ oz.	2.0
(Sanna)	1 plastic cup	2.0
CREAM OF WHEAT, cereal:		
Regular	2½ T.	22.0
*Instant	¾ cup	21.0
Mix 'n Eat, dry:		
Regular	1 packet	21.0
Baked apple & cinnamon	1 packet	29.0
Banana & spice	1 packet	29.0
Maple & brown sugar	3¾ T.	29.0
Quick	2½ T.	21.0
CREME DE BANANA LIQUEUR (Mr. Boston)	1 fl. oz.	12.0
CREME DE CACAO (Mr. Boston):		
Brown	1 fl. oz.	14.3
White	1 fl. oz.	12.0
CREME DE CAFÉ (Leroux)	1 fl. oz.	13.6
CREME DE CASSIS (Mr. Boston)	1 fl. oz.	14.1
CREME DE MENTHE:		
(Bols)	1 fl. oz.	13.0
(Hiram Walker)	1 fl. oz.	11.2
(Mr. Boston):		
Green	1 fl. oz.	16.0
White	1 fl. oz.	13.0
CREME DE NOYAUX (Mr. Boston)	1 fl. oz.	13.5

Food and Description	Measure or Quantity	Carbohydrates (grams)
CRÊPE, frozen:		
(Mrs. Paul's):		
Crab	5½-oz. pkg.	24.6
Shrimp	2½-oz. pkg.	23.8
(Stouffer's):		
Beef burgundy	6¼-oz. pkg.	24.0
Chicken with mushroom sauce	8¼-oz. pkg.	19.0
Ham & asparagus	6¼-oz. pkg.	21.0
Mushroom	6¼-oz. pkg.	27.0
CRISP RICE, cereal:		
(Ralston Purina)	1 cup	25.0
(Van Brode):		
Regular	1 cup	24.9
Cocoa	¾ cup	25.3
CRISPY WHEATS 'N RAISINS,		
cereal (General Mills)	¾ cup	23.0
CROQUETTES, frozen, seafood		
(Mrs. Paul's)	3-oz. serving	23.9
CROUTON:		
(Arnold):		
American or Danish style	½ oz.	8.7
Bavarian or English style	½ oz.	9.5
French, Italian or Mexican style	½ oz.	9.5
Croutettes (Kellogg's)	⅔ cup	14.0
CUCUMBER:		
Eaten with skin	½-lb. cucumber	7.4
Pared, 10-oz. cucumber	7½" x 1" pared	6.6
Pared	3 slices	.8
CUMIN SEED (French's)	1 tsp.	.7
CUPCAKE:		
Regular (Hostess):		
Chocolate	1 cupcake	29.8
Orange	1 cupcake	26.8
Frozen (Sara Lee) yellow	1 cupcake	31.5
*CUPCAKE MIX (Flako)	1 cupcake	25.0
CUP O' NOODLES (Nissin Foods):		
Beef	2½-oz. serving	39.2
Beef, twin pack	1.2-oz. serving	18.2
Beef onion	2½-oz. serving	36.8
Beef onion, twin pack	1.2-oz. serving	19.4
Chicken	2½-oz. serving	40.0
Chicken, twin pack	1.2-oz. serving	18.6
Pork	2½-oz. serving	40.7
Shrimp	2½-oz. serving	40.0
CURAÇAO:		
(Bols)	1 fl. oz.	10.3
(Garnier)	1 fl. oz.	12.7

Food and Description	Measure or Quantity	Carbohydrates (grams)
CURRANT, dried, Zante (Del Monte)	½ cup	47.8
CURRANT JELLY (Smucker's)	1 T.	13.5
CUSTARD:		
Chilled, *Swiss Miss*, chocolate or egg flavor	4-oz. container	22.0
Frozen (See ICE CREAM)		
*Mix, dietetic (Featherweight)	½ cup	15.0
C.W. POST, cereal:		
Family style	¼ cup	20.3
Family-style with raisins	¼ cup	20.4

D

DAIQUIRI COCKTAIL, canned (Mr. Boston) 12½% alcohol:		
Regular	3 fl. oz.	9.0
Strawberry	3 fl. oz.	12.0
DATE (Dromedary):		
Chopped	¼ cup	31.0
Pitted	5 dates	23.0
DE CHAUNAC WINE (Great Western)12% alcohol	3 fl. oz.	2.4
DELAWARE WINE (Gold Seal) 12% alcohol	3 fl. oz.	2.6
DILL SEED (French's)	1 tsp.	1.2
DING DONG (Hostess)	1 cake	21.5
DINNER, frozen (See individual listing such as BEEF, CHICKEN or ENCHILADA, etc.)		
DIP:		
Avocado (Nalley's)	1 oz.	.9
Bacon & onion (Nalley's)	1 oz.	1.1
Barbecue (Nalley's)	1 oz.	1.1
Blue cheese (Nalley's)	1 oz.	.9
Cheese-Bacon (Nalley's)	1 oz.	.8
Clam (Nalley's)	1 oz.	1.1
Cucumber & onion (Breakstone)	1 oz.	1.6
Dill pickle (Nalley's)	1 oz.	.9
Enchilada, *Fritos*	1 oz.	3.9
Garlic (Nalley's)	1 oz.	.9
Guacamole (Nalley's)	1 oz.	.9
Jalapeno:		
Fritos	1 oz.	3.7
(Hain) natural	1 oz.	2.5
(Nalley's)	1 oz.	.8

Food and Description	Measure or Quantity	Carbohydrates (grams)
Onion (Dean) French	1 oz.	2.0
Onion bean (Hain) natural	1 oz.	3.6
Ranch House (Nalley's)	1 oz.	.6
DISTILLED LIQUOR, any brand, 80, 86, 90, 94 or 100 proof	1 fl. oz.	Tr.
DOUGHNUT:		
Regular (Hostess):		
Cinnamon	1-oz. piece	14.5
Crunch	1-oz. piece	16.5
Enrobed	1-oz. piece	13.6
Old fashioned	1½-oz. piece	19.6
Powdered	1-oz. piece	15.1
Frozen (Morton):		
Bavarian creme	2-oz. piece	22.1
Boston creme	2.3-oz. piece	28.5
Chocolate iced	1½-oz. piece	19.6
Glazed	1½-oz. piece	19.2
Jelly	1.8-oz. piece	22.9
Mini	1.1-oz. piece	16.0
DRAMBUIE (Hiram Walker)	1 fl. oz.	11.0
DRUMSTICK, frozen:		
Ice cream, in a cone:		
Topped with peanuts	1 piece	22.7
Topped with peanuts & cone bisque	1 piece	23.6
Ice milk, in a cone:		
Topped with peanuts	1 piece	24.3
Topped with peanuts & cone bisque	1 piece	25.2
DUMPLING, canned (Dia-Mel) dietetic	8 oz.	28.0

E

Food and Description	Measure or Quantity	Carbohydrates (grams)
ECLAIR:		
Home recipe, with custard filling and chocolate icing	4-oz. piece	26.3
Frozen, chocolate (Rich's)	1 piece	30.0
EEL, smoked, meat only	4 oz.	0.
EGG, CHICKEN:		
Raw, white only	1 large egg	.3
Raw, yolk only	1 large egg	.1
Boiled	1 large egg	.4
Fried in butter	1 large egg	.1
Omelet, mixed with milk & cooked in fat	1 large egg	1.5

Food and Description	Measure or Quantity	Carbohydrates (grams)
Poached	1 large egg	.4
Scrambled, mixed with milk & cooked in fat	1 large egg	1.5
*EGG FOO YUNG (Chun King) stir fry	⅛ of pkg.	3.0
EGG MIX (Durkee):		
Omelet:		
*With bacon	½ of pkg.	10.0
*Puffy	½ of pkg.	11.0
Scrambled:		
Plain	.8-oz. pkg.	4.0
With bacon	1.3-oz. pkg.	6.0
EGG NOG, dairy:		
(Meadow Gold) 6% fat	½ cup	25.5
(Sealtest) 6% fat	½ cup	17.0
EGG NOG COCKTAIL, canned		
(Mr. Boston) 15% alcohol	3 fl. oz.	18.9
EGGPLANT:		
Boiled	4 oz.	4.1
Frozen:		
(Mrs. Paul's):		
Parmesan	5½-oz. serving	21.5
Slices, breaded & fried	3-oz. serving	22.4
Sticks, breaded & fried	3½-oz. serving	27.3
(Weight Watchers) parmigiana	13-oz. pkg.	25.0
EGG ROLL, frozen:		
(Chun King):		
Chicken	½-oz. roll	3.0
Meat & shrimp	½-oz. roll	3.5
Shrimp	½-oz. roll	3.8
(La Choy):		
Chicken	.4-oz. roll	3.6
Lobster	.4-oz. roll	3.6
Meat & shrimp	.2-oz. roll	2.3
Meat & shrimp	.4-oz. roll	3.5
Shrimp	.4-oz. roll	3.7
Shrimp	2½-oz. roll	14.9
EGG, SCRAMBLED & SAUSAGE, frozen (Swanson) with hashed brown potatoes, TV Brand	6½-oz. serving	22.0
EGG SUBSTITUTE:		
Egg Beaters (Fleischmann)	¼ cup	3.0
*Eggstra (Tillie Lewis)	1 egg	4.0
*Scramblers (Morningstar Farms)	1 egg	1.2
*Second Nature (Avoset)	3 T.	2.0
ELDERBERRY, without stems	4 oz.	18.6
ELDERBERRY JELLY (Smucker's)	1 T.	13.5

Food and Description	Measure or Quantity	Carbohydrates (grams)
ENCHILADA, frozen:		
Beef:		
(Banquet):		
Buffet Supper, with cheese & chili gravy	2-lb. pkg.	118.2
Dinner	12-oz. dinner	63.6
(Morton)	12-oz. dinner	47.7
(Swanson) *TV Brand*	15-oz. dinner	72.0
(Van de Kamp's):		
Dinner	12-oz. dinner	45.0
Entree, shredded	12-oz. entree	40.0
Cheese:		
(Banquet):		
Regular	12-oz. dinner	58.8
Man-Pleaser	21¼-oz. dinner	82.0
(Van de Kamp's):		
Dinner	12-oz. dinner	44.0
Entree, Ranchero	12-oz. entree	44.0
Chicken (Van de Kamp's)	7½-oz. pkg.	24.0
ENCHILADA SAUCE:		
Canned (Del Monte) hot or mild	½ cup	11.0
*Mix (Durkee)	½ cup	6.3
ENCHILADA SEASONING MIX (French's)	1⅜-oz. pkg.	20.0
ENDIVE, CURLY or ESCAROLE, cut	½ cup	1.5
EXPRESSO COFFEE LIQUEUR	1 fl. oz.	15.0

F

FARINA:		
Dry:		
(Hi-O) regular	¼ cup	33.6
Malt-O-Meal, regular	1 oz.	21.1
Malt-O-Meal, quick-cooking	1 oz.	22.0
*(Pillsbury):		
Made with milk	⅔ cup	26.0
Made with water	⅔ cup	17.0
FAT, cooking, *Crisco; Fluffo*	1 T.	0.
FENNEL SEED (French's)	1 tsp.	1.3
FIG:		
Small	1½" fig	7.7
Canned, regular pack (Del Monte) whole, solids & liq.	½ cup	28.1
Canned, dietetic pack (Featherweight) Kadota, water pack, solids & liq.	½ cup	15.0

Food and Description	Measure or Quantity	Carbohydrates (grams)
Dried, chopped	½ cup	59.1
FIG JUICE, *RealFig*	½ cup	15.8
FILBERT:		
Shelled	1 oz.	4.7
(Fisher) oil dipped, salted	½ cup	5.4
FISH AU GRATIN, frozen (Mrs. Paul's)	5-oz. serving	19.5
FISH CAKE, frozen (Mrs. Paul's):		
Breaded & fried	2-oz. cake	11.9
Thins, breaded & fried	½ of 10-oz. pkg.	30.7
FISH & CHIPS, frozen:		
(Mrs. Paul's) batter fried, light	½ of 14-oz. pkg.	43.3
(Swanson):		
TV Brand	10½-oz. dinner	38.0
TV Brand	5-oz. entree	25.0
(Van de Kamp's) batter dipped, french fried	8-oz. serving	45.0
FISH DINNER, frozen:		
(Banquet)	8¾-oz. dinner	43.6
(Mrs. Paul's):		
Au gratin	½ of 10-oz. pkg.	19.6
Parmesan	½ of 10-oz. pkg.	20.9
(Van de Kamp's) batter dipped, french fried	11-oz. dinner	39.0
(Weight Watchers) in lemon sauce, 3-compartment	13¼-oz. meal	19.1
FISH FILLET, frozen:		
(Mrs. Paul's):		
Batter fried, crunchy	2¼-oz. piece	17.2
Breaded & fried	2-oz. piece	12.0
Buttered	2½-oz. piece	.9
Miniature, batter fried	3-oz. serving	15.3
(Van de Kamp's):		
Batter dipped, french fried	3-oz. piece	12.5
Country seasoned	2.4-oz. piece	10.5
Light & crispy	2-oz. piece	10.0
FISH KABOBS, frozen:		
(Mrs. Paul's) batter fried, light	3⅓-oz. serving	17.7
(Van de Kamp's):		
Batter dipped, french fried	.4-oz. piece	1.6
Country seasoned	.4-oz. piece	1.9
FISH SANDWICH, frozen (Mrs. Paul's)		
Fillet	4⅛-oz. sandwich	23.2
FISH STICK, frozen:		
(Mrs. Paul's):		
Batter fried	1 stick	6.4

Food and Description	Measure or Quantity	Carbohydrates (grams)
Breaded & fried	1 stick	4.1
(Van de Kamp's) batter dipped, french fried	1-oz. piece	5.2
FIT 'N FROSTY (Alba '77):		
Chocolate or marshmallow flavor	1 envelope	11.0
Strawberry	1 envelope	12.0
Vanilla	1 envelope	11.3
FIVE ALIVE (Snow Crop)	6 fl. oz.	20.8
FLOUNDER:		
Baked	4 oz.	0.
Frozen:		
(Mrs. Paul's):		
Fillets, breaded & fried	2-oz. fillet	11.6
With lemon butter	4¼-oz. serving	9.4
(Weight Watchers) with lemon flavored bread crumbs	6½-oz. serving	12.0
(Weight Watchers) in Newburgh sauce	12½-oz. pkg.	11.0
FLOUR:		
Aunt Jemima, self-rising	¼ cup	23.6
Ballard, all-purpose	¼ cup	21.3
Bisquick (Betty Crocker)	¼ cup	19.0
(Elam's):		
Brown rice, whole grain	¼ cup	30.1
Buckwheat, pure	¼ cup	19.0
Rye, whole grain	¼ cup	18.2
Soy	1 oz.	8.9
Whole wheat, whole grain	1 oz.	19.8
(Featherweight):		
Gluten	¼ cup	13.7
Soy bean	¼ cup	8.2
Gold Medal (Betty Crocker):		
All purpose or unbleached	¼ cup	21.3
High protein or self-rising	¼ cup	20.3
La Pina	¼ cup	21.3
Pillsbury's Best:		
All purpose	¼ cup	21.3
Bread	¼ cup	20.1
Rye, medium	¼ cup	22.1
Sauce & gravy	1 T.	5.5
Self-rising	¼ cup	21.0
Whole wheat	¼ cup	20.0
Softasilk	¼ cup	23.0
(Swan Down) cake	¼ cup	22.0
Wondra	¼ cup	21.3
FOOD STICKS (Pillsbury) all flavors	1 stick	6.8

Food and Description	Measure or Quantity	Carbohydrates (grams)
FOUR FRUIT PRESERVE		
(Smucker's)	1 T.	13.5
FRANKEN*BERRY, cereal (General Mills)	1 cup	24.0
FRANKFURTER:		
(Best's Kosher):		
Regular	1.5-oz. frankfurter	1.5
Beef	1.5-oz. frankfurter	1.5
Cocktail	.3-oz. frankfurter	.3
Dinner	2.7-oz. frankfurter	2.7
Jumbo	2-oz. frankfurter	2.1
Mild	1.5-oz. frankfurter	1.5
(Eckrich):		
Beef or meat	1.6-oz. frankfurter	3.0
Beef or meat, jumbo	2-oz. frankfurter	3.0
Meat	1.2-oz. frankfurter	2.0
(Hormel):		
Beef	1.6-oz. frankfurter	.7
Range Brand Wrangler, smoked	1 frankfurter	.8
(Hygrade) beef, *Ball Park*	2-oz. frankfurter	<.1
(Louis Rich) turkey	1.5-oz. frankfurter	1.0
(Oscar Mayer):		
Beef	1.6-oz. frankfurter	1.4
Beef, jumbo	2-oz. frankfurter	1.2
Beef, *Big One*	4-oz. frankfurter	2.4
Little Wiener	2″ frankfurter	.2
Wiener	1.6-oz. frankfurter	1.3
Wiener with cheese	1.6-oz. frankfurter	.7
(Oscherwitz):		
Regular	1.6-oz. frankfurter	1.6
Beef	1.5-oz. frankfurter	1.5
Cocktail	.3-oz. frankfurter	.3
(Vienna) beef	1.5-oz. frankfurter	1.0
FRANKS-N-BLANKETS (Durkee)	1 piece	1.0
FRENCH TOAST, frozen (Aunt Jemima):		
Regular	1.5-oz. slice	13.2
Cinnamon swirl	1 slice	13.6
FRENCH TOAST & SAUSAGE, frozen (Swanson)	4½-oz. entree	22.0
FRITTERS, frozen (Mrs. Paul's):		
Apple	2-oz. fritter	16.1
Clam	1.9-oz. piece	14.3
Corn	2-oz. piece	15.1
Crab	1.9-oz. piece	15.3
Shrimp	½ of 7¾-oz. pkg.	27.0
Tuna	½ of 7¾-oz. pkg.	27.5

Food and Description	Measure or Quantity	Carbohydrates (grams)
FROOT LOOPS, cereal (Kellogg's)	1 cup	25.0
FROSTED RICE, cereal (Kellogg's)	1 cup	26.0
FROZEN DESSERT, dietetic (Sugarlo) any flavor	¼ pt.	14.0
FRUIT BITS, dried (Sun-Maid)	2-oz. serving	42.8
FRUIT BRUTE, cereal (General Mills)	1 cup	24.0
FRUIT COCKTAIL, canned:		
Regular pack, heavy syrup, solids & liq.:		
(Del Monte) regular & chunky	½ cup	23.0
(Libby's)	½ cup	24.7
(Stokely-Van Camp)	½ cup	23.0
Dietetic pack, solids & liq.:		
(Del Monte) *Lite*	½ cup	14.1
(Diet Delight):		
Syrup pack	½ cup	17.0
Water pack	½ cup	10.0
(Featherweight) juice pack	½ cup	12.0
(Libby's) water pack	½ cup	10.4
(S&W) *Nutradiet*:		
Juice pack	½ cup	14.0
Water pack	½ cup	10.0
(Tillie Lewis) *Tasti-Diet*	½ cup	13.5
*FRUIT COUNTRY (Comstock):		
Apple	¼ of pkg.	36.0
Blueberry	¼ of pkg.	33.0
Cherry	¼ of pkg.	38.0
Peach	¼ of pkg.	28.0
FRUIT CUP (Del Monte):		
Mixed fruits	5-oz. container	26.7
Peaches, diced	5-oz. container	27.8
FRUIT JUICE, canned (Sun-Maid)		
Purple	6 fl. oz.	25.0
FRUIT, MIXED:		
Canned (Del Monte) *Lite*	½ cup	13.6
Frozen (Birds Eye)	5-oz. serving	34.5
FRUIT PUNCH:		
Canned:		
Capri Sun	6¾ fl. oz.	25.9
(Hi-C)	6 fl. oz.	23.0
(Lincoln) party	8 fl. oz.	34.8
Chilled:		
Five Alive (Snow Crop)	6 fl. oz.	22.7
(Minute Maid)	6 fl. oz.	23.0
*Frozen, *Five Alive* (Snow Crop)	6 fl. oz.	22.7
*Mix (Hi-C)	6 fl. oz.	18.0
FRUIT ROLL (La Choy)	½-oz. roll	6.4

Food and Description	Measure or Quantity	Carbohydrates (grams)
FRUIT SALAD:		
Canned, regular pack, solids & liq.:		
(Del Monte):		
Fruits for salad	½ cup	23.0
Tropical fruit	½ cup	26.0
(Libby's) heavy syrup	½ cup	24.0
Canned, dietetic pack, solids & liq.:		
(Diet Delight)	½ cup	16.0
(Featherweight):		
Juice pack	½ cup	12.0
Water pack	½ cup	10.0
(S&W) *Nutradiet:*		
Juice pack	½ cup	14.0
Water pack	½ cup	10.0
FUDGSICLE (Popsicle Industries)	2½-fl.-oz. bar	23.0

G

Food and Description	Measure or Quantity	Carbohydrates (grams)
GARLIC:		
Flakes (Gilroy)	1 tsp.	2.6
Powder (French's)	1 tsp.	1.1
Salt (French's)	1 tsp.	1.0
GAZPACHO SOUP (Crosse & Blackwell)	6½-oz. serving	1.0
GEFILTE FISH, canned:		
(Mother's):		
Jelled, Old World	4-oz. serving	7.0
In liquid broth	4-oz. serving	7.0
(Rokeach):		
Jelled	4-oz. serving	4.0
Old Vienna	4-oz. serving	8.0
GELATIN, dry, *Carmel Kosher*	7-gram envelope	0.
GELATIN DESSERT:		
Canned, dietetic pack:		
(Dia-Mel) *Gel-A-Thin,* all flavors	4-oz. container	.2
(Estee) strawberry	4-oz. serving	11.2
*Mix:		
Regular:		
Carmel Kosher, all flavors	½ cup	20.0
(Jell-O) all flavors	½ cup	18.5
(Royal) all flavors	½ cup	19.0
Dietetic:		
Carmel Kosher	½ cup	0.
(Dia-Mel) *Gel-A-Thin*	4-oz. serving	1.0
(Estee) all flavors	½ cup	9.9

Food and Description	Measure or Quantity	Carbohydrates (grams)
(Featherweight) all flavors, artificially sweetened	½ cup	0.
(Royal) *Sweet As You Please*, all flavors	½ cup	0.
GERMAN STYLE DINNER, frozen (Swanson) *TV Brand*	11¾-oz. dinner	40.0
GINGER, powder (French's)	1 tsp.	1.2
*****GINGERBREAD MIX:**		
(Betty Crocker)	⅑ of cake	36.0
(Dromedary)	2" x 2" square	20.0
(Pillsbury)	3" square	36.0
GIN, SLOE (Mr. Boston)	1 fl. oz.	4.7
GOLDEN GRAHAMS, cereal (General Mills)	¾ cup	24.0
GOOBER GRAPE (Smucker's)	1 oz.	14.0
GOOD HUMOR (See also individual flavors)		
Chocolate chip cookie sandwich	1 piece	64.0
Chocolate eclair	3-oz. piece	25.0
Lite Fruit Stix	1.5-oz. piece	8.0
Sandwich	2.5-oz. piece	34.0
Strawberry shortcake	3-oz. piece	21.0
Toasted Almond	3-oz. piece	21.0
Vanilla, chocolate coated	3-oz. piece	12.0
Whammy, assorted	1.6-oz. piece	9.0
Whammy, chip crunch	1.6-oz. piece	10.0
GOOD N' PUDDIN (Popsicle Industries) all flavors	2¼-fl.-oz. bar	27.0
GOOSE, roasted, meat & skin	4-oz. serving	0.
GRAHAM CRAKOS, cereal (Kellogg's)	¾ cup	24.0
GRANOLA BAR, Nature Valley:		
Almond, coconut or peanut	1 bar	15.0
Cinnamon or oats 'n honey	1 bar	16.0
GRANOLA CEREAL:		
Heartland:		
Coconut	¼ cup	18.0
Plain or raisin	¼ cup	18.0
Puffs, regular or cinnamon spice	½ cup	20.0
Nature Valley:		
Cinnamon & raisin	⅓ cup	19.0
Coconut & honey	⅓ cup	18.0
Toasted oat	⅓ cup	19.0
Sun Country:		
With almonds	½ cup	34.1
With raisins	½ cup	36.9
GRANOLA CLUSTERS, *Nature Valley,* all flavors	1 roll	27.0

Food and Description	Measure or Quantity	Carbohydrates (grams)
GRAPE:		
American type (slipskin)	3½" x 3" bunch	9.9
Canned, dietetic pack (Featherweight) light, seedless, water pack	½ cup	13.0
GRAPE DRINK:		
Canned:		
(Hi-C)	6 fl. oz.	22.0
(Lincoln)	6 fl. oz.	23.9
(Welchade)	6 fl. oz.	23.0
*Frozen (Welchade)	6 fl. oz.	23.0
*Mix (Hi-C)	6 fl. oz.	17.0
GRAPEFRUIT:		
Pink & red:		
Seeded type	½ med. grapefruit	11.9
Seedless type	½ med. grapefruit	12.8
White:		
Seeded type	½ med. grapefruit	11.7
Seedless type	½ med. grapefruit	11.9
Canned, regular pack, solids & liq. (Del Monte) syrup pack	½ cup	17.5
Canned, dietetic pack, solids & liq.:		
(Del Monte) sections	½ cup	10.5
(Diet Delight) sections	½ cup	11.0
(Featherweight) sections	4-oz. serving	9.0
(S&W) *Nutradiet*, sections	½ cup	9.0
GRAPEFRUIT DRINK, canned (Lincoln)	6 fl. oz.	26.1
GRAPEFRUIT JUICE:		
Fresh, pink, red or white	½ cup	11.3
Canned, sweetened:		
(Del Monte)	6 fl. oz.	20.8
(Minute Maid)	6 fl. oz.	17.0
Canned, unsweetened:		
(Del Monte)	6 fl. oz.	16.6
(Ocean Spray)	6 fl. oz.	14.6
(Texsun)	6 fl. oz.	18.0
Chilled (Minute Maid)	6 fl. oz.	18.1
*Frozen, unsweetened (Minute Maid)	6 fl. oz.	18.3
GRAPEFRUIT JUICE COCKTAIL, canned (Ocean Spray) pink	6 fl. oz.	20.0
GRAPEFRUIT-ORANGE JUICE COCKTAIL, canned, *Musselman's*	6 fl. oz.	17.2
GRAPEFRUIT PEEL, candied	1 oz.	22.9
GRAPE JAM (Smucker's)	1 T.	13.7
GRAPE JELLY:		

Food and Description	Measure or Quantity	Carbohydrates (grams)
Sweetened:		
(Smucker's)	1 T.	13.5
(Welch's)	1 T.	13.5
Dietetic (See GRAPE SPREAD)		
GRAPE JUICE:		
Canned, unsweetened:		
(Seneca Foods)	6 fl. oz.	30.0
(Welch's)	6 fl. oz.	30.0
*Frozen:		
(Minute Maid)	6 fl. oz.	13.3
(Welch's)	6 fl. oz.	25.0
GRAPE JUICE DRINK, chilled		
(Welch's)	6 fl. oz.	27.0
GRAPE NUTS, cereal (Post):		
Flakes	¾ cup	23.0
Nuggets	¾ cup	23.4
GRAPE SPREAD, dietetic:		
(Diet Delight)	1 T.	3.0
(Estee)	1 T.	4.8
(Smucker's)	1 T.	6.0
(Welch's)	1 T.	6.2
GRAVY, canned (See also GRAVY MIX):		
Au jus (Franco-American)	2-oz. serving	2.0
Beef (Franco-American)	2-oz. serving	3.0
Brown:		
(Dawn Fresh) with mushroom broth	2-oz. serving	3.2
(Franco-American) with onion	2-oz. serving	4.0
(La Choy)	1-oz. serving	20.3
Ready Gravy	¼ cup	7.6
Chicken (Franco-American) regular or giblet	2-oz. serving	4.0
Mushroom (Franco-American)	2-oz. serving	3.0
Turkey (Franco-American)	2-oz. serving	3.0
GRAVYMASTER	1 tsp.	2.4
GRAVY WITH MEAT OR TURKEY:		
Canned (Morton House):		
Sliced beef	6¼-oz. serving	8.0
Sliced pork	6¼-oz. serving	9.0
Sliced turkey	6¼-oz. serving	7.0
Frozen:		
(Banquet):		
Giblet gravy & sliced turkey	5-oz. cooking bag	5.3
Sliced beef	2-lb. pkg.	34.5
(Green Giant):		
Sliced beef, *Toast Topper*	5-oz. serving	5.7
Sliced turkey *Toast Topper*	5-oz. serving	6.7

Food and Description	Measure or Quantity	Carbohydrates (grams)
(Swanson) sliced beef with whipped potatoes	8-oz. entree	23.0
GRAVY MIX:		
Regular:		
Au jus:		
*(Durkee)	½ cup	3.2
(Durkee) *Roastin' Bag*	1-oz. pkg.	14.0
*(French's) *Gravy Makins*	½ cup	4.0
Brown:		
*(Durkee):		
Regular	½ cup	5.0
With mushrooms	½ cup	5.5
With onions	½ cup	6.5
*(Ehler's)	½ cup	7.0
*(French's)	½ cup	6.0
*(Pillsbury)	½ cup	6.0
*(Spatini)	1-oz. serving	3.0
Chicken:		
*(Durkee)	½ cup	7.0
*(Durkee) creamy	½ cup	7.0
*(French's) *Gravy Makins*	½ cup	8.0
(Pillsbury)	½ cup	8.0
*Home style:		
(Durkee)	½ cup	5.5
(French's) *Gravy Makins*	½ cup	8.0
(Pillsbury)	½ cup	6.0
Meatloaf (Durkee) *Roastin' Bag*	1½-oz. pkg.	18.0
Mushroom:		
*(Durkee)	½ cup	5.5
*(French's) *Gravy Makins*	½ cup	6.0
Onion:		
*(Durkee)	½ cup	7.6
*(French's) *Gravy Makins*	½ cup	8.0
Pork:		
*(Durkee)	½ cup	7.0
(Durkee) *Roastin' Bag*	1½-oz. pkg.	26.0
*(French's) *Gravy Makins*	½ cup	6.0
Pot roast (Durkee) *Roastin' Bag*	1½-oz. pkg.	25.0
*Swiss steak (Durkee)	½ cup	5.3
Turkey:		
*(Durkee)	½ cup	7.0
*(French's) *Gravy Makins*	½ cup	8.0
*Dietetic (Weight Watchers):		
Brown	¼ cup	1.0
Brown, with mushrooms	¼ cup	2.0
Brown, with onion	¼ cup	2.0
Chicken	¼ cup	2.0

Food and Description	Measure or Quantity	Carbohydrates (grams)
GREENS, MIXED, canned (Sunshine)		
Solids & liq.	½ cup	2.7
GRENADINE (Garnier) no alcohol	1 fl. oz.	26.0
GUAVA	1 guava	11.7

H

Food and Description	Measure or Quantity	Carbohydrates (grams)
HADDOCK:		
Fried, breaded	4" x 3" x ½" fillet	5.8
Frozen:		
(Banquet)	8¾-oz. dinner	45.4
(Mrs. Paul's) breaded & fried	2-oz. fillet	11.8
(Swanson) filet almondine	7½-oz. entree	9.0
(Van de Kamp's) batter dipped, french fried	2-oz. piece	8.0
(Weight Watchers) with stuffing, 2-compartment	7-oz. pkg.	14.1
Smoked	4-oz. serving	0.
HALIBUT:		
Broiled	4" x 3" x ½" steak	0.
Frozen (Van de Kamp's) batter dipped, french fried	½ of 8-oz. pkg.	17.0
HAM:		
Canned:		
(Hormel):		
Chopped	¼ of 12-oz. can	.2
Chopped	¹⁄₁₆ of 8-lb. can	3.4
Chunk	6¾-oz. serving	1.5
EXL	4-oz. serving	.1
Holiday Glaze	4-oz. serving	2.5
Patties	1 patty	.4
(Oscar Mayer) *Jubilee,* extra lean, cooked	4-oz. slice	.3
(Swift):		
Hostess	3½-oz. slice	.8
Premium	1¾-oz. slice	.3
Deviled:		
(Hormel)	1-oz. serving	.1
(Libby's)	1-oz. serving	.2
(Underwood)	1 T.	Tr.
Packaged:		
(Eckrich), smoked, sliced	1-oz. slice	.7
(Hormel):		
Black peppered	.8-oz. slice	.1
Chopped	1-oz. slice	.3
Cooked	.8-oz. slice	.1
Red peppered	.8-oz. slice	.1

Food and Description	Measure or Quantity	Carbohydrates (grams)
Smoked, cooked (Oscar Mayer):	.8-oz. slice	.1
Chopped	1-oz. slice	.7
Jubilee, slice, boneless	8-oz. slice	0.
Jubilee, steak, boneless, 95% fat free	2-oz. steak	0.
Smoked, cooked	1-oz. slice	0.
HAMBURGER (See *McDONALD'S* and *BURGER KING*)		
HAMBURGER MIX:		
*Hamburger Helper (General Mills):		
Beef noodle	⅕ of pkg.	25.0
Beef Romanoff	⅕ of pkg.	28.0
Cheeseburger	⅕ of pkg.	28.0
Chili tomato	⅕ of pkg.	29.0
Hash	⅕ of pkg.	24.0
Lasagna	⅕ of pkg.	33.0
Pizza	⅕ of pkg.	33.0
Potato Stroganoff	⅕ of pkg.	28.0
Rice Oriental	⅕ of pkg.	35.0
Spaghetti	⅕ of pkg.	31.0
Stew	⅕ of pkg.	23.0
Make A Better Burger (Lipton) mildly seasoned or onion	⅓ oz.	5.0
HAMBURGER SEASONING MIX:		
**(Durkee)	1 cup	7.5
(French's)	1-oz. pkg.	20.0
HAM & BUTTER BEAN SOUP (Campbell) *Chunky*	10¾-oz. can	34.0
HAM & CHEESE:		
(Hormel) loaf	1-oz. slice	.3
(Oscar Mayer):		
Loaf	1-oz. slice	.6
Spread	⅙ of 6-oz. tube	.7
HAM DINNER, frozen:		
(Banquet)	10-oz. dinner	47.7
(Morton)	10-oz. dinner	56.9
(Swanson) *TV Brand*	10¼-oz. dinner	47.0
HAM SALAD, canned (Carnation)	1½-oz. serving	3.4
HAM SALAD SPREAD (Oscar Mayer)	1-oz. serving	3.0
HAWAIIAN PUNCH:		
Canned:		
Cherry	6 fl. oz.	22.9
Grape	6 fl. oz.	23.4
Orange	6 fl. oz.	24.4
Red	6 fl. oz.	21.3

75

Food and Description	Measure or Quantity	Carbohydrates (grams)
Very berry	6 fl. oz.	21.6
*Mix, red punch	8 fl. oz.	25.0
HEADCHEESE (Oscar Mayer)	1-oz. serving	0.
HERRING, canned (Vita):		
Bismarck, drained	5-oz. jar	6.9
Cocktail, drained	8-oz. jar	24.8
In cream sauce	8-oz. jar	18.1
Matjes, drained	8-oz. jar	26.2
Tastee Bits, drained	8-oz. jar	24.7
HERRING, SMOKED, kippered	4-oz. serving	0.
HICKORY NUT, shelled	1 oz.	3.6
HOMINY GRITS:		
Dry:		
(Albers)	1½ oz.	33.0
(Aunt Jemima)	3 T.	22.5
(Quaker):		
Regular	3 T.	22.4
Instant	.8-oz. packet	17.7
Instant, with imitation bacon bits or cheese flavored	1-oz. packet	21.6
(3-Minute Brand) quick	⅛ cup	22.2
Cooked	1 cup	27.0
HONEY, strained	1 T.	16.5
HONEYCOMB, cereal (Post)	1⅓ cups	25.1
HONEYDEW	2" x 7" wedge	7.2
HOPPING JOHN (Green Giant)	⅓ pkg.	16.7
HORSERADISH:		
Raw, pared	1 oz.	5.6
Prepared (Gold's)	1-oz. serving	.4

I

Food and Description	Measure or Quantity	Carbohydrates (grams)
ICE CREAM & FROZEN CUSTARD (See also listing by flavor or brand name or FROZEN DESSERT)		
(Dean) 10.4% fat	1 cup	41.1
ICE CREAM CONE, cone only (Comet):		
Regular cone	1 piece	4.0
Rolled sugar	1 piece	9.0
ICE CREAM CUP (Comet) cup only	1 cup	4.0
ICE MILK:		
Hardened	¼ pt.	14.6
Soft-serve	¼ pt.	19.6
(Meadow Gold):		
Chocolate, *Viva*	½ cup	18.0
Vanilla, *Viva*	½ cup	17.0

Food and Description	Measure or Quantity	Carbohydrates (grams)
(Swift) *Light 'n Easy*, all flavors	½ cup	17.0
ITALIAN DINNER, frozen		
(Banquet)	11-oz. dinner	44.6

J

JAM, sweetened or dietetic (See JAM or PRESERVE or JAM, individual flavors)		
JELLY, sweetened (See also individual flavors) (Crosse & Blackwell) all flavors	1 T.	12.8
JERUSALEM ARTICHOKE, pared	4 oz.	18.9
JOHANNISBERG RIESLING:		
(Deinhard)	3 fl. oz.	4.5
(Inglenook)	3 fl. oz.	.9

K

KABOOM, cereal (General Mills)	1 cup	23.0
KALE:		
Boiled, leaves only	4 oz.	6.9
Canned (Sunshine) chopped, solids & liq.	½ cup	2.8
Frozen:		
(Birds Eye) chopped	⅓ of pkg.	5.0
(McKenzie) chopped	⅓ of pkg.	4.5
(Seabrook Farms) chopped	⅓ of pkg.	4.5
(Southland) chopped	⅛ of 16-oz. pkg.	5.0
KARO SYRUP (See SYRUP)		
KEFIR (Alta-Dena Dairy):		
Plain	1 cup	13.0
Flavored	1 cup	24.0
KIDNEY:		
Beef, braised	4 oz.	.9
Calf, raw	4 oz.	.1
Lamb, raw	4 oz.	1.0
KIELBASA:		
(Eckrich) skinless	2-oz. serving	2.0
(Hormel)	3-oz. serving	1.2
(Vienna)	2-oz. serving	1.1
KING VITAMAN, cereal (Quaker)	1¼ cups	23.2
KIRSCH, liqueur (Garnier)	1 fl. oz.	8.8
KIX, cereal (General Mills)	1½ cups	24.0

77

Food and Description	Measure or Quantity	Carbohydrates (grams)
KNOCKWURST (Best's Kosher; Oscherwitz):		
Regular	3-oz. piece	3.0
Beef	3-oz. piece	2.9
***KOOL AID** (General Foods):		
Unsweetened	8 fl. oz.	25.0
Pre-sweetened, all flavors but tropical punch	8 fl. oz.	23.2
Pre-sweetened, tropical punch	8 fl. oz.	24.5
KUMQUAT, flesh & skin	5 oz.	19.4

L

Food and Description	Measure or Quantity	Carbohydrates (grams)
LAKE COUNTRY, wine (Taylor)		
Gold, 12% alcohol	3 fl. oz.	5.4
LAMB	Any quantity	0.
LASAGNA:		
Canned:		
(Hormel) *Short Orders*	7½-oz. can	24.0
(Nalley's)	8-oz. serving	25.0
Frozen:		
(Green Giant):		
With meat sauce, *Bake 'n Serve*	7-oz. serving	27.8
With meat sauce, boil-in-bag	9-oz. cooking bag	32.2
(Hormel) beef	10-oz. serving	30.4
(Stouffer's)	10½-oz. serving	35.8
(Swanson):		
Hungry Man, with meat	12¾-oz. entree	51.0
Hungry Man, with meat	17¾-oz. dinner	91.0
TV Brand	13-oz. dinner	54.0
(Weight Watchers)	13-oz. meal	35.1
Mix (Golden Grain) *Stir-N-Serv*	⅛ of 7-oz. pkg.	25.9
LEEKS	4 oz.	12.7
LEMON:		
Whole	2⅛″ lemon	11.7
Peeled	2⅛″ lemon	6.1
LEMONADE:		
Canned:		
Capri Sun	6¾ fl. oz.	23.3
Country Time	6 fl. oz.	16.7
(Hi-C)	6 fl. oz.	17.0
Chilled (Minute Maid) regular or pink	6 fl. oz.	18.0
***Frozen:**		
Country Time, regular or pink	6 fl. oz.	17.0
(Minute Maid)	6 fl. oz.	19.6

Food and Description	Measure or Quantity	Carbohydrates (grams)
(Sunkist)	6 fl. oz.	21.1
*Mix:		
Country Time, regular or pink	6 fl. oz.	16.5
(Hi-C)	6 fl. oz.	19.0
Kool-Aid, sweetened, regular or pink	6 fl. oz.	18.8
Kool-Aid, unsweetened, regular or pink	6 fl. oz.	16.7
Lemon Tree (Lipton)	6 fl. oz.	16.5
(Minute Maid) regular or pink	6 fl. oz.	20.0
LEMON EXTRACT (Virginia Dare)	1 tsp.	0.
LEMON JUICE:		
Canned, ReaLemon	1 T.	.8
Frozen (Minute Maid) unsweetened	1 fl. oz.	2.2
*LEMON-LIMEADE DRINK, mix (Minute Maid)	6 fl. oz.	20.0
LEMON PEEL, CANDIED	1 oz.	22.9
LEMON & PEPPER SEASONING (French's)	1 tsp.	1.0
LENTIL SOUP, canned (Crosse & Blackwell) with ham	½ of 13-oz. can	13.0
LETTUCE:		
Bibb or Boston	4" head	4.1
Cos or Romaine, shredded or broken into pieces	½ cup	.8
Grand Rapids, Salad Bowl or Simpson	2 large leaves	1.8
Iceberg, New York or Great Lakes	¼ of 4¾" head	3.3
LIEBFRAUMILCH WINE:		
(Anheuser)	3 fl. oz.	.9
(Deinhard)	3 fl. oz.	3.6
LIFE, cereal (Quaker) regular or cinnamon	⅔ cup	19.7
LIME, peeled	2" dia.	4.9
*LIMEADE, frozen (Minute Maid)	6 fl. oz.	20.1
LIME JUICE, ReaLime	1 T.	.5
LINGUINI IN CLAM SAUCE, frozen:		
(Ronzoni)	4-oz. serving	16.0
(Stouffer's)	½ of 10½-oz. pkg.	35.8
LITCHI NUT, fresh, flesh only	4 oz.	18.6
LIVER:		
Beef:		
Fried	6½" x 2⅜" x ⅜" slice	4.5
(Swift) cooked	3.2-oz. serving	3.1

Food and Description	Measure or Quantity	Carbohydrates (grams)
Calf, fried	6½" x 2⅜" x ⅜" slice	3.4
Chicken, simmered	2" x 2" x ⅝" liver	.8
LIVERWURST SPREAD (Underwood)	1-oz. serving	1.3
LOBSTER:		
Cooked, meat only	1 cup	.4
Canned, meat only	4 oz.	.3
Frozen, South African lobster tail:		
3 in 8-oz. pkg.	1 piece	.2
4 in 8-oz. pkg.	1 piece	.1
5 in 8-oz. pkg.	1 piece	<.1
LOBSTER NEWBURG	1 cup	12.8
LOBSTER PASTE, canned	1 oz.	.4
LOBSTER SALAD	4 oz.	2.6
LOBSTER SOUP, cream of (Crosse & Blackwell)	6½-oz. serving	6.5
LOG CABIN SYRUP (See SYRUP)		
LOQUAT, fresh, flesh only	2 oz.	17.0
LUCKY CHARMS, cereal (General Mills)	1 cup	24.0
LUNCHEON MEAT (See also individual listings such as BOLOGNA, etc.):		
(Oscar Mayer)	1-oz. slice	.4
Banquet loaf (Eckrich)	1-oz. slice	1.5
Bar-B-Q Loaf (Oscar Mayer) 90% fat free	1-oz. slice	1.4
BBQ Loaf (Hormel)	1-oz. slice	.5
Beef honey roll sausage (Oscar Mayer) 90% fat free	.8-oz. slice	.7
Beef, jellied (Hormel) loaf	1.2-oz. slice	0.
Buffet loaf (Hormel)	1-oz. slice	.5
Gourmet loaf (Eckrich)	1-oz. slice	1.7
Ham & cheese (See HAM & CHEESE)		
Ham roll sausage (Oscar Mayer)	.8-oz. slice	.5
Honey loaf:		
(Eckrich)	1-oz. slice	1.8
(Hormel)	1-oz. slice	.6
(Oscar Mayer) 95% fat free	1-oz. slice	1.1
Liver cheese (Oscar Mayer) pork fat wrapped	1.3-oz. slice	.2
Liver loaf (Hormel)	1-oz. slice	.6
Luxury loaf (Oscar Mayer) 95% fat free	1-oz. slice	1.5
Meat loaf	1 oz.	.9

Food and Description	Measure or Quantity	Carbohydrates (grams)
New England brand sliced sausage:		
(Hormel)	1-oz. slice	.2
(Oscar Mayer) 92% fat free	1-oz. slice	.6
Old fashioned loaf:		
(Eckrich)	1-oz. slice	2.0
(Oscar Mayer)	1-oz. slice	2.3
Olive loaf:		
(Hormel)	1-oz. slice	1.5
(Oscar Mayer)	1-oz. slice	2.8
Peppered beef (Vienna)	1-oz. serving	.4
Peppered loaf:		
(Hormel)	1-oz. serving	.4
(Oscar Mayer) 93% fat free	1-oz. slice	1.3
Pickle loaf:		
(Eckrich)	1-oz. slice	1.5
(Hormel)	1-oz. slice	1.3
Pickle & pimiento loaf (Oscar Mayer)	1-oz. slice	3.0
Picnic loaf (Oscar Mayer)	1-oz. slice	1.6
Spiced (Hormel)	1-oz. serving	.5

M

Food and Description	Measure or Quantity	Carbohydrates (grams)
MACADAMIA NUT (Royal Hawaiian)	1 oz.	4.6
MACARONI:		
Cooked:		
8-10 minutes, firm	1 cup	39.1
14-20 minutes, tender	1 cup	32.3
Canned (Franco-American) Pizz Os	7½-oz. can	34.0
MACARONI & BEEF:		
Canned, in tomato sauce:		
(Franco-American) Beefy Os	7½-oz. can	29.0
(Nalley's)	8-oz. serving	29.5
Frozen:		
(Banquet)	12-oz. dinner	55.1
(Banquet) Buffet Supper	2-lb. pkg.	106.4
(Green Giant)	9-oz. entree	30.7
(Stouffer's)	11½-oz. pkg.	39.8
(Swanson) TV Brand	12-oz. dinner	55.0
MACARONI & CHEESE:		
Canned:		
(Franco-American):		
Regular	7⅜-oz. can	24.0
Cheese Os	7½-oz. can	21.0
Elbow	7⅜-oz. can	23.0

Food and Description	Measure or Quantity	Carbohydrates (grams)
(Hormel) *Short Orders*	7½-oz. can	22.0
Frozen:		
(Banquet) *Buffet Supper*	2-lb. pkg.	110.9
(Banquet) dinner	12-oz. dinner	45.6
(Green Giant)	9-oz. cooking bag	35.8
(Green Giant) oven bake	6-oz. serving	23.7
(Morton)	8-oz. casserole	36.4
(Stouffer's)	12-oz. pkg.	47.8
(Swanson)	12-oz. entree	40.0
(Swanson) *TV Brand*	12½-oz. dinner	55.0
(Van de Kamp's)	10-oz. pkg.	46.0
Mix:		
(Golden Grain) deluxe	¼ of 7¼-oz. pkg.	38.1
*(Pennsylvania Dutch Brand)	½ cup	25.0
*(Prince)	¾ cup	34.6
MACARONI & CHEESE PIE, frozen (Swanson)	7-oz. pie	26.0
MACARONI SALAD, canned (Nalley's)	4-oz. serving	15.9
MACE (French's)	1 tsp.	.8
MACKEREL, Atlantic, broiled, with fat	8½" x 2½" x ½" fillet	0.
MADEIRA WINE (Leacock)	3 fl. oz.	6.3
MAI TAI COCKTAIL, canned (Mr. Boston) 12½% alcohol	3 fl. oz.	12.3
MALTED MILK MIX (Carnation):		
Chocolate	3 heaping tsps.	18.0
Natural	3 heaping tsps.	15.6
MALT LIQUOR, *Champale,* regular	12 fl. oz.	12.2
MALT-O-MEAL, cereal:		
Regular	1 T.	7.3
Chocolate	1 T.	7.0
MANDARIN ORANGE (See TANGERINE)		
MANGO, fresh	1 med. mango	22.5
MANHATTAN COCKTAIL:		
Canned (Mr. Boston) 20% alcohol	3 fl. oz.	6.3
Mix:		
Dry (Bar-Tender's)	1 serving	5.6
Liquid, canned (Holland House)	1½ fl. oz.	10.5
MARGARINE:		
Regular	1 pat (1" x 1.3" x 1", 5 grams)	.1
(Parkay) regular, soft or squeeze	1 T.	.1
MARGARINE, IMITATION OR DIETETIC:		
(Parkay)	1 T.	0.

Food and Description	Measure or Quantity	Carbohydrates (grams)
(Weight Watchers)	1 T.	0.
MARGARINE, WHIPPED (Blue Bonnet; Miracle; Parkay)	1 T.	0.
MARGARITA COCKTAIL:		
Canned (Mr. Boston):		
Regular, 12½% alcohol	3 fl. oz.	10.8
Strawberry, 12½% alcohol	3 fl. oz.	18.9
Mix:		
Dry (Bar-Tender's)	1 serving	17.3
Liquid (Holland House)	1½ fl. oz.	14.2
MARINADE MIX:		
Chicken (Adolph's)	1-oz. packet	14.4
Meat:		
(Adolph's)	.8-oz. pkg.	8.5
(Durkee)	1-oz. pkg.	9.0
(French's)	1-oz. pkg.	16.0
MARJORAM (French's)	1 tsp.	.8
MARMALADE:		
Sweetened:		
(Ann Page)	1 T.	14.8
(Keiller)	1 T.	15.0
(Smucker's)	1 T.	13.5
Dietetic:		
(Dia-Mel)	1 T.	0.
(Featherweight)	1 T.	4.0
(Louis Sherry)	1 T.	0.
(Smucker's) imitation	1 T.	6.0
(S&W) *Nutradiet*	1 T.	3.0
(Tillie Lewis) *Tasti-Diet*	1 T.	3.0
MARSHMALLOW FLUFF	1 heaping tsp.	14.4
MARTINI COCKTAIL:		
Canned, gin (Mr. Boston) extra dry, 20% alcohol	3 fl. oz.	0.
Canned, vodka (Mr. Boston) 20% alcohol	3 fl. oz.	.9
Mix, liquid (Holland House)	2 fl. oz.	5.1
MASA HARINA (Quaker)	⅓ cup	27.4
MASA TRIGO (Quaker)	⅓ cup	24.7
MATZO, dietetic (Horowitz Margareten)	1 matzo	26.0
MAYONNAISE:		
Real (Hellmann's)	1 T.	.1
Dietetic or imitation:		
(Diet Delight) *Mayo-Lite*	1 T.	Tr.
(Featherweight) *Soyamaise*	1 T.	0.
(Tillie Lewis) *Tasti-Diet,* *Maylonaise*	1 T.	1.0
(Weight Watchers)	1 T.	1.0

Food and Description	Measure or Quantity	Carbohydrates (grams)
MAYPO, cereal:		
30-second	¼ cup	16.4
Vermont-style	¼ cup	22.0
McDONALD'S:		
Big Mac	1 sandwich	40.6
Biscuit:		
Ham	1 biscuit	43.0
Sausage	1 biscuit	42.5
Cheeseburger	1 hamburger	29.8
Chicken McNuggets	1 serving	17.6
Cookie:		
Chocolate Chip	1 package	44.8
McDonaldland	1 package	48.7
Egg McMuffin	1 serving	31.0
Egg, scrambled	1 serving	2.5
English muffin, with butter	1 muffin	29.5
Filet-O-Fish	1 sandwich	37.4
Grapefruit juice	6 fl. oz.	17.9
Hamburger	1 hamburger	29.5
Hotcakes with butter & syrup	1 serving	93.9
McChicken	1 sandwich	39.8
McFeast	1 serving	31.3
McRib	1 sandwich	43.7
Orange juice	6 fl. oz.	19.6
Pie:		
Apple	1 pie	29.3
Cherry	1 pie	32.1
Potato:		
Fried	1 regular order	26.1
Hash brown	1 order	14.0
Quarter Pounder	1 hamburger	32.7
Quarter Pounder, with cheese	1 hamburger	32.2
Sausage, pork	1 serving	.6
Shake:		
Chocolate	1 serving	65.5
Strawberry	1 serving	62.1
Vanilla	1 serving	59.6
Sundae:		
Caramel	1 sundae	52.5
Hot fudge	1 sundae	46.2
Strawberry	1 sundae	46.1
MEATBALL DINNER or ENTREE, frozen (Swanson) *TV Brand*	9¼-oz. entree	26.0
MEATBALL SEASONING MIX:		
*(Durkee) Italian style	1 cup	4.5
(French's)	¼ of 1½-oz. pkg.	7.0
*MEATBALL SOUP, canned (Campbell) alphabet	10-oz. serving	16.0

Food and Description	Measure or Quantity	Carbohydrates (grams)
MEATBALL STEW, canned:		
Dinty Moore	7½-oz. serving	15.1
(Morton House)	8-oz. serving	18.0
(Nalley's)	8-oz. serving	18.2
MEATBALL, SWEDISH, frozen		
(Stouffer's) with noodles	11-oz. pkg.	32.8
MEAT LOAF DINNER, frozen:		
(Banquet):		
Regular	11-oz. dinner	29.0
Man-Pleaser	19-oz. dinner	63.6
(Morton):		
Regular	11-oz. dinner	28.1
Country Table	15-oz. dinner	59.7
(Swanson):		
TV Brand	10¾-oz. dinner	48.0
TV Brand	9-oz. entree	30.0
MEAT LOAF SEASONING MIX		
(French's)	1½-oz. pkg.	40.0
MEAT, POTTED:		
(Hormel)	1-oz. serving	.4
(Libby's)	1-oz. serving	.3
MEAT TENDERIZER (French's)		
regular or seasoned	1 tsp.	Tr.
MELBA TOAST, salted (Old London):		
Garlic, onion or white rounds	1 piece	1.8
Pumpernickel, rye, wheat or white	1 piece	3.4
Sesame, flat	1 piece	3.0
MELON BALL, in syrup, frozen	½ cup	18.2
MEXICAN DINNER, frozen:		
(Banquet) combination	12-oz. dinner	72.1
(Swanson) TV Brand, combination	16-oz. dinner	75.0
(Van de Kamp's) combination	11-oz. dinner	49.0
MILK, CONDENSED, Dime Brand; Eagle Brand; Magnolia Brand	1 T.	9.5
MILK, DRY, non-fat instant:		
*(Alba)	1 cup	11.6
*(Alba) chocolate flavor	1 cup	12.9
*(Pet)	8 fl. oz.	12.0
*(Sanalac)	8 fl. oz.	11.0
MILK, EVAPORATED:		
Regular:		
(Carnation)	1 fl. oz.	3.0
(Pet)	1 fl. oz.	3.1
Filled:		
Dairymate	½ cup	12.0
(Pet)	½ cup	12.0
Low fat (Carnation)	1 fl. oz.	3.0

Food and Description	Measure or Quantity	Carbohydrates (grams)
Skimmed:		
(Carnation)	1 fl. oz.	3.5
Pet 99	1 fl. oz.	3.5
MILK, FRESH:		
Buttermilk (Friendship)		12.
Chocolate (Dairylea)		
Low fat, *Viva*, 3% fat, vitamins A & D	1 cup	12.0
Skim (Dairylea; Meadow Gold)	1 cup	11.0
Whole (Dairylea; Meadow Gold)	1 cup	11.0
MILK, GOAT, whole	1 cup	11.2
MILNOT, dairy vegetable blend	1 fl. oz.	3.1
MINESTRONE SOUP, canned:		
(Campbell):		
Chunky	9½-oz. can	21.0
*Condensed	10-oz. serving	13.0
(Crosse & Blackwell)	6½-oz. serving	18.0
MINI-WHEATS, cereal (Kellogg's) any flavor	1 biscuit	6.0
MINT LEAVES	½ oz.	.8
MOLASSES:		
(Brer Rabbit) dark	1 T.	10.6
(Grandma's) unsulphured	1 T.	15.0
MORTADELLA, sausage	1-oz. serving	.2
MOSELLE WINE (Great Western)	3 fl. oz.	2.9
MOST, cereal (Kellogg's)	½ cup	22.0
MOUSSE, canned, dietetic (Featherweight) chocolate	½ cup	14.0
MUFFIN:		
Regular, plain	1.4-oz. muffin	16.9
Blueberry:		
(Morton) frozen:		
Regular	1.6-oz. muffin	22.9
Rounds	1½-oz. muffin	20.9
Bran (Arnold) *Orowheat*	2.3-oz. muffin	30.0
Corn:		
(Morton) frozen:		
Regular	1.7-oz. muffin	20.3
Rounds	1½-oz. muffin	20.9
(Thomas')	2-oz. muffin	25.8
English:		
(Arnold)	2.3-oz. muffin	30.0
(Pepperidge Farm):		
Regular	1 muffin	27.0
Cinnamon raisin	1 muffin	28.0
Roman Meal	2⅓-oz. muffin	29.8
(Thomas') regular or frozen	2-oz. muffin	25.9
Raisin (Arnold) *Orowheat*	2.5-oz. muffin	35.0

Food and Description	Measure or Quantity	Carbohydrates (grams)
Sourdough (Wonder)	2-oz. muffin	27.3
MUFFIN MIX:		
Blueberry:		
*(Betty Crocker) wild	1 muffin	19.0
(Duncan Hines)	1/12 of pkg.	17.0
Bran (Duncan Hines)	1/12 of pkg.	.3
Corn:		
*(Betty Crocker)	1 muffin	25.0
*(Dromedary)	1 muffin	20.0
*(Flako)	1 muffin	23.0
MUG-O-LUNCH (General Mills):		
Chicken flavored noodles & sauce	1 pouch	25.0
Macaroni & cheese sauce	1 pouch	41.0
Noodles & beef flavored sauce	1 pouch	30.0
Spaghetti & tomato sauce	1 pouch	31.0
MULLIGAN STEW, canned, *Dinty Moore, Short Orders*	7½-oz. can	14.0
MUSCATEL WINE (Gallo) 14% alcohol	3 fl. oz.	7.9
MUSHROOM:		
Raw, whole	½ lb.	9.7
Raw, trimmed, slices	½ cup	1.5
Canned:		
(Green Giant)	2-oz. serving	1.7
(Shady Oaks)	4-oz. can	2.0
Frozen (Green Giant) whole, in butter sauce	3-oz. serving	2.6
MUSHROOM, CHINESE, dried	1 oz.	18.9
MUSHROOM SOUP, canned:		
Regular pack:		
*(Ann Page) cream of	1 cup	10.2
*(Campbell):		
Cream of	10-oz. serving	11.0
Cream of, *Soup For One*	7½-oz. can	13.0
Golden	10-oz. serving	11.0
(Crosse & Blackwell) cream of	6½-oz. serving	8.0
*(Rokeach) cream of, prepared with milk	10-oz. serving	20.0
Dietetic:		
(Campbell) cream of, low sodium	7½-oz. can	10.0
*(Dia-Mel) cream of	8-oz. serving	9.0
MUSHROOM SOUP MIX:		
Carmel Kosher	6 fl. oz.	2.0
*(Lipton):		
Beef	8 oz.	7.0
Cream of, *Cup-A-Soup*	6 fl. oz.	10.0
MUSSEL, in shell	1 lb.	7.2

Food and Description	Measure or Quantity	Carbohydrates (grams)
MUSTARD:		
Powder (French's)	1 tsp.	.3
Prepared:		
Brown (French's)	1 tsp.	.3
Horseradish (Nalley's)	1 tsp.	.3
Onion (French's)	1 tsp.	1.6
Salad (French's) cream	1 tsp.	.3
Yellow (Gulden's)	1 tsp.	.4
MUSTARD GREENS:		
Canned (Sunshine) solids & liq.	½ cup	3.2
Frozen:		
(Birds Eye)	⅓ of pkg.	3.0
(McKenzie)	⅓ of pkg.	3.4
(Seabrook Farms)	⅓ of pkg.	3.4
(Southland)	⅕ of 16-oz. pkg.	3.0

N

Food and Description	Measure or Quantity	Carbohydrates (grams)
NATURAL CEREAL:		
Heartland, any flavor	¼ cup	18.0
(Quaker):		
Hot, whole wheat	⅓ cup	21.8
100%	¼ cup	17.4
100%, with apple & cinnamon or raisins & dates	¼ cup	18.0
NATURE SNACKS (Sun-Maid):		
Carob Crunch	1 oz.	16.8
Raisin Crunch	1 oz.	19.7
Rocky Road	1 oz.	19.1
Tahitian Treat	1 oz.	19.4
Yogurt crunch	1 oz.	19.7
NECTARINE, flesh only	4 oz.	19.4
NOODLE:		
Dry (Pennsylvania Dutch Brand) any type	1 oz.	20.0
Cooked, 1½" strips	1 cup	37.3
NOODLES & BEEF:		
Canned (Hormel) *Short Orders*	7½-oz. can	15.0
Frozen (Banquet) *Buffet Supper*	2-lb. pkg.	83.6
NOODLE, CHOW MEIN:		
(Chun King)	⅛ of 5-oz. can	13.0
(La Choy):	½ cup	16.8
NOODLE MIX:		
*(Betty Crocker):		
Almondine	¼ of pkg.	27.0
Romanoff	¼ of pkg.	23.0
Stroganoff	¼ of pkg.	26.0

Food and Description	Measure or Quantity	Carbohydrates (grams)
Noodle Roni, parmesano *(Lipton)	⅛ of 6-oz. pkg.	22.5
Egg Noodles & Sauce:		
Beef	½ cup	26.0
Butter	½ cup	24.0
Cheese	½ cup	24.0
Chicken	½ cup	25.0
Side Quicks (General Mills):		
Noodles & beef or cheese sauce	¼ of pkg.	21.0
Noodles & butter sauce	¼ of pkg.	20.0
Noodles & chicken sauce	¼ of pkg.	19.0
*NOODLE, RAMEN (La Choy) canned:		
Beef	½ of 3-oz. can	27.6
Chicken	½ of 3-oz. can	27.6
Oriental	½ of 3-oz. can	27.7
NOODLE, RICE (La Choy)	1 oz.	20.6
NOODLE ROMANOFF, frozen (Stouffer's)	⅓ of pkg.	15.9
*NOODLE SOUP, canned (Campbell):		
Curly with chicken	10-oz. serving	11.0
& ground beef	10-oz. serving	14.0
NUT, MIXED:		
Dry roasted:		
(A&P)	1 oz.	6.6
(Flavor House)	1 oz.	5.4
(Planters)	1 oz.	7.0
Oil roasted:		
(Excel) with peanuts	1 oz.	5.4
(Planters) with or without peanuts	1 oz.	6.0
NUTMEG (French's)	1 tsp.	.9
*NUT*Os* (General Mills)	1 T.	3.0
NUTRI-GRAIN, cereal (Kellogg's):		
Barley	⅔ cup	23.0
Corn	½ cup	24.0
Rye or wheat	⅔ cup	24.0
NUTRIMATO, canned (Mott's)	6 fl. oz.	17.0

O

OAT FLAKES, cereal (Post)	⅔ cup	20.1
OATMEAL:		
(H-O):		
Regular, old fashioned	1 T.	2.6

Food and Description	Measure or Quantity	Carbohydrates (grams)
Instant:		
Regular, boxed	1 T.	2.6
Regular, packets	1-oz. packet	17.9
With bran & spice	1½-oz. packet	29.0
With cinnamon & spice	1⅝-oz. packet	33.6
With country apple & brown sugar	1.1-oz. packet	22.7
With maple & brown sugar flavor	1½-oz. packet	31.8
Sweet & mellow	1.4-oz. packet	28.7
Quick, old fashioned	½ cup	22.2
(Quaker):		
Regular, old fashioned	½ cup	18.4
Instant:		
Regular	1-oz. packet	18.1
Apple & cinnamon	1¼-oz. packet	26.0
Bran & raisin	1½-oz. packet	29.2
Cinnamon & spice	1⅝-oz. packet	24.8
Maple & brown sugar	1½-oz. packet	31.9
Raisin & spice	1½-oz. packet	31.4
Quick	⅓ cup	18.4
*(Ralston Purina):		
Regular	½ cup	22.2
Quick	⅓ cup	18.0
(3-Minute Brand) Stir 'n Eat:		
Dutch apple brown sugar	1⅛-oz. packet	23.3
Natural flavor	1-oz. packet	18.0
OIL, SALAD or COOKING	Any quantity	0.
OKRA, frozen:		
(Birds Eye) whole	⅓ of pkg.	7.0
(McKenzie) cut	⅓ of pkg.	6.1
(Seabrook Farms) whole	⅓ of pkg.	6.9
(Southland) cut	⅕ of 16-oz. pkg.	5.0
OLIVE:		
Green	4 med. or 3 extra large or 2 giant	.2
Ripe, Mission	3 small or 2 large	.3
ONION:		
Raw	2½" onion	8.7
Boiled, pearl onion	½ cup	6.0
Canned (Durkee) O & C:		
Boiled	1-oz. serving	2.0
Creamed	1-oz. serving	17.0
Dehydrated flakes (Gilroy)	1 tsp.	1.2
Frozen:		
(Birds Eye):		
Chopped	⅓ of pkg.	2.0
Creamed	⅓ of pkg.	11.0

Food and Description	Measure or Quantity	Carbohydrates (grams)
Whole	⅓ of pkg.	10.0
(Green Giant) creamed	⅓ of pkg.	5.1
(Mrs. Paul's) french-fried rings	½ of 5-oz. pkg.	21.2
(Southland) chopped	⅕ of 10-oz. pkg.	5.0
ONION BOUILLON:		
(Croydon House)	1 tsp.	2.3
(Herb-Ox)	1 cube	1.3
MBT	1 packet	2.0
ONION, GREEN	1 small onion	.9
ONION SEASONING, SALAD		
(French's)	1 T.	3.0
ONION SOUP, canned:		
(Campbell):		
Regular	10-oz. serving	11.0
Cream of, made with water	10-oz. serving	15.0
Cream of, made with water and milk	10-oz. serving	20.0
(Crosse & Blackwell)	6½-oz. serving	4.8
ONION SOUP MIX:		
Carmel Kosher	6 fl. oz.	2.4
(Lipton):		
Regular	1 cup	6.0
Beefy	1 cup	4.0
Cup-A-Soup	1 pkg.	5.0
ORANGE:		
Peeled	½ cup	16.0
Sections	4 oz.	9.0
ORANGEADE, chilled (Sealtest)	½ cup	8.0
ORANGE-APRICOT JUICE COCKTAIL, *Musselman's*	6 fl. oz.	20.5
ORANGE DRINK:		
Canned:		
Capri Sun	6¾-fl.-oz. can	26.1
(Hi-C)	6 fl. oz.	23.0
(Lincoln)	6 fl. oz.	23.9
*Mix (Hi-C)	6 fl. oz.	17.0
ORANGE EXTRACT (Virginia Dare)	1 tsp.	0.
***ORANGE-GRAPEFRUIT JUICE,** frozen (Minute Maid)	6 fl. oz.	19.1
ORANGE JUICE:		
Canned:		
(Del Monte):		
Unsweetened	6 fl. oz.	18.5
Sweetened	6 fl. oz.	17.4
(Sunkist) unsweetened	½ cup	14.0
(Texsun) sweetened	6 fl. oz.	20.0

Food and Description	Measure or Quantity	Carbohydrates (grams)
Chilled (Minute Maid)	6 fl. oz.	19.7
*Frozen:		
Bright & Early, imitation	6 fl. oz.	21.6
(Minute Maid)	6 fl. oz.	20.5
(Sunkist)	6 fl. oz.	21.7
ORANGE-PINEAPPLE DRINK, canned (Lincoln)	8 fl. oz.	32.4
ORANGE-PINEAPPLE JUICE, canned (Texsun)	6 fl. oz.	21.0
ORANGE-PINEAPPLE JUICE COCKTAIL, canned, *Musselman's*	6 fl. oz.	20.5
***ORANGE PLUS** (Birds Eye)	6 fl. oz.	23.5
ORANGE SPREAD, dietetic (Estee)	1 tsp.	1.9
OREGANO (French's)	1 tsp.	1.0
OVALTINE, chocolate flavor	¾-oz. serving	17.9
OYSTER:		
Raw:		
Eastern	19-31 small or 13-19 med.	8.2
Pacific & Western	6-9 small or 4-6 med.	15.4
Canned (Bumble Bee) solids & liq.	1 cup	15.4
Fried	4-oz. serving	21.1
OYSTER STEW, home recipe	½ cup	5.7
***OYSTER STEW SOUP,** canned (Campbell):		
Made with milk	10-oz. serving	12.0
Made with water	10-oz. serving	5.0

P

***PANCAKE BATTER,** frozen (Aunt Jemima):		
Plain	4″ pancake	14.1
Blueberry	4″ pancake	13.8
Buttermilk	4″ pancake	14.2
PANCAKE & SAUSAGE, frozen (Swanson)	6-oz. entree	50.0
***PANCAKE & WAFFLE MIX:**		
Plain:		
(Aunt Jemima):		
Original	4″ pancake	12.7
Complete	4″ pancake	8.5
(Log Cabin) complete	4″ pancake	8.7
(Pillsbury) *Hungry Jack:*		
Complete, bulk	4″ pancake	12.3
Complete, packets	4″ pancake	11.6
Extra Lights	4″ pancake	9.3

Food and Description	Measure or Quantity	Carbohydrates (grams)
Panshakes	4″ pancake	13.3
Blueberry (Pillsbury) *Hungry Jack*	4″ pancake	14.0
Buckwheat (Aunt Jemima)	4″ pancake	8.3
Buttermilk:		
(Aunt Jemima):		
Original	4″ pancake	13.3
Complete	4″ pancake	15.3
(Betty Crocker) complete	4″ pancake	13.7
(Pillsbury) *Hungry Jack*,		
complete	4″ pancake	9.7
Whole wheat (Aunt Jemima)	4″ pancake	10.7
Dietetic (Tillie Lewis) complete,		
Tasti-Diet	4″ pancake	8.7
PANCAKE & WAFFLE SYRUP		
(See SYRUP)		
PAPAYA, fresh:		
Cubed	½ cup	9.1
Juice	4 oz.	18.8
PAPRIKA (French's)	1 tsp.	1.1
PARSLEY:		
Fresh, chopped	1 T.	.3
Dried (French's)	1 tsp.	.6
PASSION FRUIT, giant, whole	1 lb.	11.3
PASTINA (Ann Page)	1 oz.	20.5
PASTRAMI:		
(Eckrich) sliced	1-oz. serving	1.3
(Vienna)	1-oz. serving	0.
PASTRY SHELL, frozen		
(Pepperidge Farm)	1 shell	15.0
PÂTÉ:		
De foie gras	1 T.	.7
Liver (Hormel)	1 T.	.3
PDQ:		
Chocolate	1 T.	14.8
Strawberry	1 T.	15.1
PEA, green:		
Fresh, boiled	½ cup	9.9
Canned, regular pack, solids & liq.:		
(Del Monte):		
Early	½ cup	9.9
Seasoned	½ cup	9.8
(Festal) sweet, tiny	½ cup	9.0
(Green Giant):		
Early, with onions	½ cup	10.6
Sweet	½ cup	8.5
Sweetlets	½ cup	8.2
Sweet, with onion	½ cup	8.5

Food and Description	Measure or Quantity	Carbohydrates (grams)
(Kounty Kist):		
Early	½ cup	12.8
Sweet	½ cup	8.5
(Le Sueur) early	½ cup	9.3
(Libby's) sweet	½ cup	11.6
(Lindy) sweet	½ cup	12.8
(Stokely-Van Camp) early	½ cup	12.5
Canned, dietetic pack, solids & liq.:		
(Diet Delight)	½ cup	8.0
(Featherweight) sweet	½ cup	12.0
(S&W) *Nutradiet*	½ cup	8.0
Frozen:		
(Birds Eye):		
In cream sauce	⅓ of pkg.	13.7
With sliced mushrooms	⅓ of pkg.	10.7
Sweet	⅓ of pkg.	12.0
(Green Giant):		
Creamed, *Bake 'n Serve*	⅓ of pkg.	11.2
Early, small	4-oz. serving	12.5
Sweet	4½-oz. serving	14.1
Sweet, in butter sauce	⅓ of pkg.	8.1
(McKenzie) petite	⅓ of pkg.	10.3
(Seabrook Farms)	⅓ of pkg.	13.1
(Seabrook Farms) petite	⅓ of pkg.	10.3
PEA & CARROT:		
Canned, regular pack, solids & liq.:		
(Del Monte)	½ cup	9.4
(Libby's)	½ cup	10.3
Canned, dietetic pack, solids & liq.		
(Diet Delight)	½ cup	6.0
Frozen (Birds Eye)	⅓ of pkg.	8.7
PEA & CAULIFLOWER, frozen		
(Birds Eye) creamed	⅓ of pkg.	11.9
PEA, CROWDER, frozen		
(Southland)	⅕ of 16-oz. pkg.	21.0
PEA & ONION, frozen (Birds Eye)	⅓ of pkg.	11.7
PEA POD:		
Fresh, boiled, drained	4-oz. serving	10.8
Frozen (La Choy)	6-oz. pkg.	20.4
PEA & POTATO, frozen (Birds Eye)		
in cream sauce	⅓ of pkg.	16.3
PEA SOUP, GREEN:		
*Canned, regular pack (Campbell)	11-oz. serving	34.0
Canned, dietetic pack (Campbell)		
low sodium	7½-oz. can	24.0
*Mix (Lipton)	1 cup	22.0

Food and Description	Measure or Quantity	Carbohydrates (grams)
PEA SOUP, SPLIT:		
Canned:		
(Campbell):		
Chunky, with ham	19-oz. can	58.0
*Condensed, with ham & bacon	11-oz. serving	32.0
(Grandma Brown's)	8-oz. serving	28.2
*Frozen (Mother's Own)	8-oz. serving	20.0
PEACH:		
Fresh, with thin skin	2″ peach	9.6
Fresh, slices	½ cup	8.2
Canned, regular pack, solids & liq.:		
(Del Monte):		
Cling	½ cup	22.8
Spiced	½ cup	20.6
(Libby's):		
Halves in heavy syrup	½ cup	25.4
Sliced in heavy syrup	½ cup	24.7
(Stokely-Van Camp)	½ cup	24.5
Canned, dietetic pack, solids & liq.:		
(Del Monte) *Lite,* Cling	½ cup	12.6
(Diet Delight):		
Cling, syrup pack	½ cup	14.0
Cling, water pack	½ cup	7.0
(Featherweight):		
Juice pack	½ cup	12.0
Water pack	½ cup	8.0
(S&W) *Nutradiet:*		
Juice pack	½ cup	14.0
Water pack	½ cup	8.0
Dried, canned (Del Monte)	2-oz. serving	35.2
Frozen (Birds Eye) sliced	5-oz. serving	34.1
PEACH FRUIT DRINK (Hi-C):		
Canned	6 fl. oz.	23.0
*Mix	6 fl. oz.	18.0
PEACH PRESERVE or JAM:		
Sweetened (Smucker's):	1 T.	13.5
Dietetic:		
(Dia-Mel)	1 T.	0.
(Featherweight)	1 T.	4.0
(Featherweight) artificially sweetened	1 T.	1.0
PEACH SPREAD, dietetic (Tillie Lewis) *Tasti Diet*	1 T.	3.0
PEANUT:		
Dry roasted:		
(Fisher) unsalted	1 oz.	5.0

Food and Description	Measure or Quantity	Carbohydrates (grams)
(Frito-Lay)	1 oz.	6.2
(Planters)	1 oz.	5.4
Oil roasted (Planters)	1 oz. (jar)	5.0
PEANUT BUTTER:		
Regular pack:		
(Elam's) natural with defatted wheat germ	1 T.	2.1
(Jif) creamy	1 T.	2.7
(Peter Pan) crunchy or smooth	1 T.	3.1
(Planters) creamy or crunchy	1 T.	3.0
(Skippy):		
Creamy	1 T.	3.0
Super chunk	1 T.	2.9
(Smucker's) creamy, crunchy or natural	1 T.	3.0
Low sodium:		
(Peter Pan)	1 T.	2.3
(S&W) *Nutradiet*	1 T.	2.0
PEANUT BUTTER BAKING CHIPS		
(Reese's)	3 T. (1 oz.)	12.8
PEA PUREE, dietetic (Featherweight)	1 cup	29.0
PEAR:		
Whole	3" x 2½" pear	25.4
Canned, regular pack:		
(Del Monte)	½ cup	21.3
(Libby's)	½ cup	25.1
Canned, dietetic pack:		
(Del Monte) *Lite*	½ cup	13.8
(Featherweight):		
Juice pack	½ cup	15.0
Water pack	½ cup	10.0
(S&W) *Nutradiet:*		
Juice pack	½ cup	15.0
Water pack	½ cup	10.0
PEBBLES, cereal:		
Cocoa	⅞ cup	24.2
Fruity	⅞ cup	24.4
PECAN:		
Halves	67 pieces	1.0
Dry roasted:		
(Fisher)	1 oz.	4.5
(Planters)	1 oz.	5.0
PEP, cereal (Kellogg's)	¾ cup	23.0
PEPPER:		
Black (French's)	1 tsp.	1.5
Lemon (Durkee)	1 tsp.	.2

Food and Description	Measure or Quantity	Carbohydrates (grams)
Seasoned (Lawry's)	1 tsp.	1.6
PEPPER, CHILI, canned:		
(Del Monte):		
Green, whole	½ cup	5.0
Jalapeno, whole	½ cup	6.0
Yellow, whole	½ cup	4.0
Old El Paso, green, chopped or whole	1 oz.	1.4
(Ortega):		
Diced, strips or whole	1 oz.	1.1
Jalapeno, diced or whole	1 oz.	1.7
PEPPERONI:		
(Hormel) sliced	1-oz. serving	.3
(Swift)	1-oz. serving	1.0
PEPPER & ONION, frozen		
(Southland):		
Diced	2 oz.	3.0
Red & green	2 oz.	4.0
*PEPPER POT SOUP, canned (Campbell)	10-oz. serving	11.0
PEPPER STEAK, frozen:		
*(Chun King) stir fry	⅛ of pkg.	3.0
(Stouffer's)	½ of 10½-oz. pkg.	34.9
PEPPER, STUFFED:		
Home recipe	2¾" x 2½" pepper with 1⅛ cups stuffing	31.1
Frozen:		
(Green Giant)	7-oz. serving	18.1
(Weight Watchers) with veal	11¾-oz. meal	22.0
PEPPER, SWEET:		
Green, whole	1 med.	2.9
Red, whole	1 med.	2.4
Frozen (Southland) green or red & green	2 oz.	3.0
PERCH:		
White, meat only	4 oz.	0.
Yellow, meat only	4 oz.	0.
Frozen:		
(Banquet)	8¾-oz. dinner	49.8
(Mrs. Paul's) fillets, breaded & fried	2-oz. fillet	8.8
(Van de Kamp's) batter dipped, french fried	2.3-oz. piece	10.0
(Weight Watchers) with lemon-flavored bread crumbs	6½-oz. serving	11.0
PERNOD (Julius Wile)	1 fl. oz.	1.1

Food and Description	Measure or Quantity	Carbohydrates (grams)
PERSIMMON	4.4-oz. fruit	20.7
PICKLE:		
Cucumber, fresh or bread & butter:		
(Fanning's)	1 fl. oz.	3.3
(Featherweight) no salt added	1 fl. oz.	3.0
(Nalley's) chips	1 oz.	6.5
Dill:		
(Featherweight) whole, low sodium	1 oz.	1.0
(Nalley's) regular or Polish style	1 oz.	.6
(Smucker's):		
Candied sticks	4" stick	11.0
Hamburger, sliced	1 slice	0.
Polish, whole	3½" pickle	1.0
Spears	3½" long spear	1.0
Hamburger (Nalley's) chips	1 oz.	.6
Kosher dill:		
(Claussen) whole	1.9-oz. pickle	1.2
(Featherweight) no salt added	1 fl. oz.	1.0
(Nalley's)	2-oz. serving	1.7
(Smucker's):		
Baby	2¾" long	.5
Whole	3½" long	1.0
Sweet:		
(Nalley's):		
Regular	1 oz.	10.5
Nubbins	1 oz.	7.9
(Smucker's):		
Candied mix	1 piece	3.3
Gherkins	2" long pickle	3.5
Whole	2½" long pickle	4.0
Sweet 'n sour (Claussen) slices	1 slice	.8
PIE:		
Regular, commercial type, not frozen:		
Apple:		
Home recipe, two-crust	⅛ of 9" pie	60.2
(Hostess)	4½-oz. pie	53.7
Banana, home recipe, cream or custard	⅛ of 9" pie	46.7
Berry (Hostess)	4½-oz. pie	51.1
Blackberry, home recipe, two-crust	⅛ of 9" pie	54.4
Blueberry, home recipe, two-crust	⅛ of 9" pie	55.1
Boston cream, home recipe	½ of 8" pie	34.3

Food and Description	*Measure or Quantity*	*Carbohydrates (grams)*
Cherry:		
Home recipe, two-crust	1/6 of 9" pie	60.7
(Hostess)	4½-oz. pie	58.8
Chocolate chiffon, home recipe	1/6 of 9" pie	61.2
Chocolate meringue, home recipe	1/6 of 9" pie	46.9
Coconut custard, home recipe	1/6 of 9" pie	37.8
Lemon (Hostess)	4½-oz. pie	52.4
Mince, home recipe, two-crust	1/6 of 9" pie	65.1
Peach (Hostess)	4½-oz. pie	52.4
Pecan (Frito-Lay's)	3-oz. serving	53.5
Pumpkin, home recipe, one-crust	1/6 of 9" pie	37.3
Raisin, home recipe, two-crust	1/6 of 9" pie	67.9
Rhubarb, home recipe, two-crust	1/6 of 9" pie	60.4
Frozen:		
Apple:		
(Banquet)	1/5 of 20-oz. pie	42.6
(Morton):		
Regular	1/6 of 24-oz. pie	40.9
Great Little Desserts	8-oz. pie	88.6
Great Little Desserts, Dutch	7.8-oz. pie	95.3
(Sara Lee)	1/6 of 31-oz. pie	43.2
(Sara Lee) Dutch	1/6 of 30-oz. pie	50.6
Banana cream:		
(Banquet)	1/6 of 14-oz. pie	19.9
(Morton):		
Regular	1/6 of 16-oz. pie	19.7
Great Little Desserts	3½-oz. pie	25.8
Blueberry:		
(Banquet)	1/6 of 20-oz. pie	37.5
(Morton):		
Regular	1/6 of 24-oz. pie	38.6
Great Little Desserts	8-oz. pie	86.4
(Sara Lee)	1/6 of 31-oz. pie	44.8
Cherry:		
(Banquet)	1/6 of 20-oz. pie	33.8
(Morton):		
Regular	1/6 of 24-oz. pie	42.0
Great Little Desserts	8-oz. pie	86.4
(Sara Lee)	1/6 of 31-oz. pie	48.0
Chocolate cream:		
(Banquet)	1/6 of 14-oz. pie	21.8
(Morton):		
Regular	1/6 of 16-oz. pie	22.8
Great Little Desserts	3½-oz. pie	28.8
Coconut cream:		
(Banquet)	1/6 of 14-oz. pie	19.0

Food and Description	Measure or Quantity	Carbohydrates (grams)
(Morton):		
Regular	⅙ of 16-oz. pie	22.0
Great Little Desserts	3½-oz. pie	28.8
Coconut custard:		
(Banquet)	⅙ of 20-oz. pie	28.3
(Morton) *Great Little Desserts*	6½-oz. pie	53.5
Custard (Banquet)	⅙ of 20-oz. pie	38.1
Lemon cream:		
(Banquet)	⅙ of 14-oz. pie	21.8
(Morton):		
Regular	⅙ of 16-oz. pie	22.0
Great Little Desserts	3½-oz. pie	27.8
Mince:		
(Banquet)	⅙ of 20-oz. pie	38.5
(Morton)	⅙ of 24-oz. pie	45.5
Neapolitan (Morton)	⅙ of 16-oz. pie	23.0
Peach:		
(Banquet)	⅙ of 20-oz. pie	35.8
(Morton)	⅙ of 24-oz. pie	38.7
(Sara Lee)	⅙ of 31-oz. pie	56.2
Pumpkin:		
(Banquet)	⅙ of 20-oz. pie	32.3
(Morton)	⅙ of 24-oz. pie	36.4
(Sara Lee)	⅛ of 45-oz. pie	49.4
Strawberry cream:		
(Banquet)	⅙ of 14-oz. pie	22.5
(Morton)	⅙ of 16-oz. pie	22.0
PIE CRUST, frozen (Banquet)		
9″ shell:		
Regular	1 crust	61.9
Deep dish	1 crust	78.8
PIE CRUST MIX:		
(Betty Crocker):		
Regular	1/16 of pkg.	10.0
Stick	⅛ of stick	10.0
*(Flako)	⅙ of 9″ pie crust	25.2
*(Pillsbury) mix or stick	⅙ of two-crust pie	27.0
PIE FILLING (See also PUDDING or PIE FILLING):		
Apple (Comstock)	⅙ of 21-oz. can	24.0
Apple rings or slices (See APPLE, canned)		
Apricot (Comstock)	⅙ of 21-oz. can	24.0
Banana cream (Comstock)	⅙ of 21-oz. can	22.0
Blueberry (Comstock)	⅙ of 21-oz. can	26.0
Cherry (Comstock)	⅙ of 21-oz. can	27.0
Chocolate cream (Comstock)	⅙ of 21-oz. can	27.0

Food and Description	Measure or Quantity	Carbohydrates (grams)
Coconut cream (Comstock)	⅙ of 21-oz. can	24.0
Coconut custard, home recipe, made with egg yolk and milk	5-oz. serving (including crust)	41.3
Lemon (Comstock)	⅙ of 21-oz. can	33.0
Mincemeat (Comstock)	⅙ of 21-oz. can	36.0
Peach (Comstock)	⅙ of 21-oz. can	27.0
Pineapple (Comstock)	⅙ of 21-oz. can	25.0
Pumpkin (See also PUMPKIN, canned) (Comstock)	⅙ of 27-oz. can	38.0
Raisin (Comstock)	⅙ of 21-oz. can	30.0
Strawberry (Comstock)	⅙ of 21-oz. can	28.0
***PIE MIX**, Boston cream (Betty Crocker)	⅛ of pie	48.0
PIEROGIES, frozen (Mrs. Paul's):		
Cabbage	5-oz. serving	64.0
Potato & cheese	5-oz. serving	56.6
Sauerkraut, Polish-style	5-oz. serving	60.2
PIGS FEET, pickled	4-oz. serving	0.
PIMIENTO, canned, drained:		
(Dromedary)	1-oz. serving	2.0
(Ortega)	¼ cup	1.3
(Sunshine) diced or sliced	1 T.	.9
PIÑA COLADA:		
Canned (Mr. Boston) 12½% alcohol	3 fl. oz.	34.2
Mix, dry (Party Tyme)	½-oz. pkg.	16.0
Mix, liquid (Holland House)	2 fl. oz.	30.0
PINEAPPLE:		
Fresh, chunks	½ cup	13.7
Canned, regular pack, solids & liq.:		
(Del Monte) syrup pack:		
Crushed	½ cup	22.7
Slices, medium	½ cup	22.4
Tidbits	½ cup	22.9
(Dole):		
Juice pack	½ cup	17.5
Syrup pack	½ cup	24.7
Canned, dietetic or unsweetened, solids & liq.:		
(Del Monte):		
Chunks, juice pack	½ cup	16.8
Slices, juice pack	½ cup	19.6
(Diet Delight) juice pack	½ cup	18.0
(Featherweight):		
Juice pack	½ cup	18.0
Water pack	½ cup	15.0
(S&W) *Nutradiet*, sliced	1 slice	7.5

Food and Description	*Measure or Quantity*	*Carbohydrates (grams)*
PINEAPPLE-GRAPEFRUIT JUICE DRINK, canned:		
(Del Monte)	6 fl. oz.	23.7
(Dole) pink	6 fl. oz.	25.4
(Texsun)	6 fl. oz.	22.0
PINEAPPLE JUICE:		
Canned, unsweetened:		
(Del Monte)	6 fl. oz.	26.2
(Dole)	6 fl. oz.	25.4
(Texsun)	6 fl. oz.	24.0
*Frozen (Minute Maid)	6 fl. oz.	22.7
PINEAPPLE-ORANGE DRINK, canned (Hi-C)	6 fl. oz.	23.0
PINEAPPLE-ORANGE JUICE:		
Canned (Del Monte)	6 fl. oz.	24.0
*Frozen (Minute Maid)	6 fl. oz.	23.0
PINEAPPLE PRESERVE or JAM, sweetened (Smucker's)	1 T.	13.7
PINE NUT, pignolias, shelled	1 oz.	3.3
PINOT CHARDONNAY WINE (Paul Masson) 12% alcohol	3 fl. oz.	2.4
PISTACHIO NUT:		
In shell	½ cup	6.3
Shelled	¼ cup	5.9
(Fisher) roasted, shelled, salted	1 oz.	5.4
PIZZA PIE:		
Regular, not frozen:		
Home recipe	⅛ of 14" pie	21.2
(Pizza Hut):		
Cheese	½ of 10" pie	53.2
Pepperoni	½ of 10" pie	54.4
Supreme	½ of 10" pie	54.4
Frozen:		
Canadian style bacon (Celeste)	8-oz. pie	50.4
Cheese:		
(Celeste)	½ of 7-oz. pie	28.6
(Celeste)	¼ of 19-oz. pie	36.2
(La Pizzeria):		
Regular	¼ of 20-oz. pie	33.0
Thick crust	⅓ of 18½-oz. pie	46.0
(Stouffer's) French Bread	½ of 10½-oz. pkg.	42.8
Totino's	½ of pie	53.0
(Weight Watchers)	6-oz. pie	31.0
Combination:		
(Celeste) Chicago style	¼ of 24-oz. pie	36.2
Totino's, classic	⅓ of pie	48.0
(Van de Kamp's) thick crust	¼ of 23.4-oz. pie	24.0
(Weight Watchers) deluxe	7¼-oz. pie	27.9

Food and Description	Measure or Quantity	Carbohydrates (grams)
Deluxe:		
(Celeste)	½ of 9-oz. pie	31.3
(Celeste)	¼ of 23½-oz. pie	33.9
(Stouffer's) French Bread	½ of 12⅜-oz. pkg.	45.7
Hamburger (Stouffer's) French Bread	½ of 12¼-oz. pkg.	37.8
Mexican style (Van de Kamp's)	½ of 11-oz. pie	27.0
Pepperoni:		
(Celeste)	½ of 7¼-oz. pie	27.1
(Celeste)	¼ of 20-oz. pie	34.8
(Stouffer's) French Bread	½ of 11¼-oz. pkg.	43.8
Totino's	½ of pie	52.0
(Van de Kamp's) thick crust	¼ of 22-oz. pie	38.0
Sausage:		
(Celeste)	½ of 8-oz. pie	29.8
(Celeste)	¼ of 22-oz. pie	34.7
(Stouffer's) French Bread	½ of 12-oz. pkg.	43.8
Totino's:		
Regular	½ of pie	54.0
Deep crust	⅙ of pie	33.0
(Weight Watchers)	6¾-oz. pie	29.1
Sausage & mushroom:		
(Celeste)	½ of 9-oz. pie	28.4
(Celeste)	¼ of 24-oz. pie	34.1
(Stouffer's) French Bread	½ of 12½-oz. pie	39.8
Sicilian style (Celeste) deluxe	¼ of 26-oz. pie	45.4
Suprema (Celeste):		
Regular	½ of 10-oz. pie	26.1
Without meat	½ of 8-oz. pie	24.6
Vegetable (Weight Watchers)	7¼-oz. pie	35.0
Mix:		
Regular (Jeno's)	½ of pkg.	62.0
Cheese:		
(Jeno's)	½ of pkg.	62.0
Skillet Pizza (General Mills)	¼ of pkg.	30.0
Pepperoni:		
(Jeno's)	½ of pkg.	67.0
Skillet Pizza (General Mills)	¼ of pkg.	31.0
Sausage, *Skillet Pizza* (General Mills)	¼ of pkg.	29.0
PIZZA SAUCE, canned:		
(Contadina)	8-oz. serving	23.0
(Ragu)	5-oz. serving	15.0
PIZZA SEASONING SPICE (French's)	1 tsp.	1.0
PLUM:		
Fresh, Japanese & hybrid	2" plum	6.9
Fresh, halves, prune-type	½ cup	15.8

Food and Description	Measure or Quantity	Carbohydrates (grams)
Canned, regular pack (Stokely-Van Camp)	½ cup	30.0
Canned, dietetic pack, solids & liq.:		
(Diet Delight) purple, juice pack	½ cup	18.6
(Featherweight) purple:		
Juice pack	½ cup	18.0
Water pack	½ cup	9.0
(S&W) *Nutradiet*, juice pack	½ cup	20.0
PLUM JELLY, dietetic (Featherweight)	1 T.	4.0
PLUM PRESERVE or JAM (Smucker's)	1 T.	13.5
P.M. FRUIT DRINK, canned (Mott's)	6 fl. oz.	22.0
POLYNESIAN-STYLE DINNER, frozen (Swanson) *TV Brand*	13-oz. dinner	65.0
POMEGRANATE, whole	1 lb.	41.7
POMMARD WINE (B&G)	3 fl. oz.	.4
POPCORN:		
*Plain, home made:		
(Jiffy Pop)	½ of 5-oz. pkg.	29.8
(Pillsbury) microwave popcorn	1 cup	5.5
Packaged:		
Buttered (Old London)	1 cup	6.4
Caramel-coated:		
(Bachman)	1-oz. serving	23.0
(Old London):		
Without peanuts	1¾-oz. bag	43.6
With peanuts	1 cup	30.2
With cheese	¾-oz. bag	6.6
Cheese flavored (Bachman)	1-oz. serving	14.0
Cracker Jack	¾-oz. serving	16.7
*POPOVER MIX (Flako)	1 popover	25.0
POPPY SEED (French's)	1 tsp.	.8
POPSICLE, twin pop	3-fl.-oz. pop	17.0
POP TARTS (See TOASTER PASTRY OR CAKE)		
PORK:		
Fresh	Any quantity	0.
Loin	Any quantity	0.
Cured ham	Any quantity	0.
PORK DINNER, frozen (Swanson) *TV Brand*	11¼-oz. dinner	48.0
PORK RINDS, *Baken-ets*	1 oz.	1.0
PORK STEAK, BREADED, frozen (Hormel)	3-oz. serving	11.0
PORK, SWEET & SOUR, frozen:		
(Chun King)	½ of 15-oz. pkg.	26.0

104

Food and Description	Measure or Quantity	Carbohydrates (grams)
(La Choy)	½ of 15-oz. pkg.	45.2
PORT WINE:		
(Gallo)	3 fl. oz.	7.8
(Great Western) Solera	3 fl. oz.	11.5
(Louis M. Martini)	3 fl. oz.	2.0
*POSTUM, instant	6 fl. oz.	2.0
POTATO:		
Fresh, cooked:		
Au gratin	½ cup	17.9
Baked, peeled	2½" dia. potato	20.9
Boiled, peeled	4.2-oz. potato	17.7
French fried	10 pieces	20.5
Hash browned, home recipe	½ cup	28.4
Mashed, milk & butter added	½ cup	12.1
Canned:		
(Del Monte) drained	1 cup	28.4
(Sunshine) whole, solids & liq.	1 cup	20.9
Frozen:		
(Birds Eye):		
Crinkle cuts	3-oz. serving	18.4
French fries	3-oz. serving	16.8
Tasti Puffs	¼ of 10-oz. pkg.	18.0
Tiny Taters	⅕ of 16-oz. pkg.	22.0
(Green Giant):		
Au gratin, Bake 'n Serve	⅓ of 10-oz. pkg.	12.1
Diced, in sour cream sauce	1 cup	36.0
Stuffed with cheese-flavored topping	5-oz. entree	30.0
(McKenzie) whole, boiled	3½-oz. serving	14.9
(Ore-Ida):		
Crispers	3.2-oz. serving	27.7
Golden Crinkles	3.2-oz. serving	21.0
Golden Fries	3.2-oz. serving	23.4
Hash browns, Southern style, with butter sauce	3-oz. serving	15.0
Shoestrings	3.3-oz. serving	27.5
Whole, small, peeled	3.2-oz. serving	17.1
(Seabrook Farms) whole, boiled	3½-oz. serving	14.9
(Southland) whole	4-oz. serving	16.0
(Stouffer's):		
Au gratin	⅓ of pkg.	12.9
Scalloped	⅓ of pkg.	13.9
POTATO & BACON, canned (Hormel) *Short Orders,* au gratin	7½-oz. can	20.0
POTATO & BEEF, canned, *Dinty Moore, Short Orders,* hashed	7½-oz. can	25.0
POTATO CHIP:		
(Bachman) any flavor	1 oz.	14.0

105

Food and Description	Measure or Quantity	Carbohydrates (grams)
(Frito-Lay's)	1 oz.	15.1
Lay's	1 oz.	14.0
Lay's, sour cream & onion flavor	1 oz.	15.0
(Nalley's)	1 oz.	14.2
(Planters) stackable	1 oz.	17.0
Pringle's:		
Regular	1 oz.	11.9
Light	1 oz.	16.8
POTATO & HAM, canned (Hormel)		
Short Orders, scalloped	7½-oz. can	18.0
*POTATO MIX:		
Au gratin:		
(Betty Crocker)	½ cup	21.0
(French's) *Big Tate*	½ cup	23.0
Creamed (Betty Crocker)	½ cup	20.0
Hash browns:		
(Betty Crocker) with onion	½ cup	22.0
(French's) *Big Tate*	½ cup	22.0
Julienne (Betty Crocker)	½ cup	18.0
Mashed:		
American Beauty	½ cup	16.0
(Betty Crocker) *Buds*	½ cup	15.0
(French's) *Big Tate*	½ cup	16.0
(Pillsbury) *Hungry Jack*, flakes	½ cup	17.0
Scalloped:		
(Betty Crocker)	½ cup	18.0
(French's) *Big Tate*	½ cup	25.0
Sour cream & chives (Betty Crocker)	½ cup	18.0
*POTATO PANCAKE MIX		
(French's) *Big Tate*	3″ pancake	5.7
POTATO SALAD:		
Home recipe	½ cup	16.8
Canned (Nalley's):		
Regular	4-oz. serving	17.0
German style	4-oz. serving	18.2
*POTATO SOUP (Campbell):		
Made with water	10-oz. serving	14.0
Made with water and milk	10-oz. serving	17.0
POTATO STICK (Durkee) *O & C*	1½-oz. can	22.0
POUND CAKE (See CAKE, Pound)		
PRALINES 'N CREAM ICE CREAM		
(Baskin-Robbins)	1 scoop (2½ fl. oz.)	23.7
PRESERVES (See also individual listing under flavor):		
(Ann Page) all flavors	1 T.	9.6
(Crosse & Blackwell)	1 T.	14.8

Food and Description	Measure or Quantity	Carbohydrates (grams)
PRETZEL:		
(Bachman) regular or butter	1 oz.	21.0
(Nabisco) *Mister Salty*, Dutch	1 piece	11.0
(Old London) nuggets	1 oz.	22.5
(Pepperidge Farm):		
Nuggets or sticks	1¼ oz.	26.3
Twist, tiny	1 oz.	21.6
(Rokeach) *Baldies*	1 oz.	20.0
PRODUCT 19, cereal (Kellogg's)	¾ cup	24.0
PRUNE:		
Dried, cooked	8 prunes & 5 T. liq.	66.1
Canned:		
Regular pack (Sunsweet)	5-6 prunes	32.9
Dietetic (Featherweight)		
stewed, water pack	½ cup	35.0
PRUNE JUICE, canned:		
(Del Monte)	6 fl. oz.	33.2
(Mott's):		
Regular	6 fl. oz.	34.0
With prune pulp	6 fl. oz.	30.0
(Sunsweet) regular	6 fl. oz.	33.0
PRUNE NECTAR (Mott's)	6 fl. oz.	25.0
PRUNE WHIP, home recipe	½ cup	24.9
PUDDING or PIE FILLING:		
Canned, regular pack:		
Banana (Del Monte)	5-oz. container	30.1
Butterscotch (Del Monte)	5-oz. container	30.8
Chocolate:		
(Betty Crocker)	5-oz. serving	30.0
(Del Monte)	5-oz. container	33.0
(Hunt's) *Snack Pack*	5-oz. container	28.0
Lemon (Hunt's) *Snack Pack*	5-oz. container	32.0
Rice:		
(Betty Crocker)	½ cup	25.0
(Comstock)	½ of 7½-oz. can	23.0
(Hunt's) *Snack Pack*	5-oz. container	27.0
(Menner's)	½ of 7½-oz. can	23.0
Tapioca:		
(Betty Crocker)	½ cup	22.0
(Del Monte)	5-oz. container	30.1
(Hormel) *Short Orders*	5-oz. container	23.0
Vanilla:		
(Betty Crocker)	5-oz. serving	29.0
(Del Monte)	5-oz. container	32.1
(Hormel) *Short Orders*	5-oz. container	29.0
Canned, dietetic (Sego) all flavors	4-oz. serving	19.5
Chilled, *Swiss Miss*:		
Butterscotch	4-oz. container	22.0

Food and Description	Measure or Quantity	Carbohydrates (grams)
Chocolate	4-oz. container	25.0
Tapioca	4-oz. container	22.0
Vanilla	4-oz. container	24.0
Frozen (Rich's):		
Banana	3-oz. container	19.3
Butterscotch	4½-oz. container	27.4
Chocolate	4½-oz. container	27.1
Vanilla	4½-oz. container	27.5
*Mix, sweetened, regular and instant:		
Banana:		
(Jell-O):		
Regular	⅛ of 9″ pie, excluding crust	18.0
Cream, instant	½ cup	13.0
(Royal):		
Regular	½ cup	27.0
Instant	½ cup	29.0
Butter pecan (Jell-O) instant	½ cup	29.0
Butterscotch:		
(Jell-O) regular or instant	½ cup	30.0
(My-T-Fine) regular	½ cup	38.0
(Royal):		
Regular	½ cup	27.0
Instant	½ cup	29.0
Chocolate:		
(Jell-O):		
Regular	½ cup	29.0
Instant	½ cup	34.0
(My-T-Fine):		
Regular	½ cup	27.0
Regular, fudge	½ cup	27.0
(Royal):		
Regular	½ cup	33.0
Instant	½ cup	35.0
Coconut:		
(Jell-O) regular, cream	⅛ of 8″ pie, excluding crust	17.0
(Royal) instant	½ cup	30.0
Coffee (Royal) instant	½ cup	29.0
Custard:		
Jell-O Americana, egg, golden	½ cup	24.0
(Royal) regular	½ cup	22.0
Flan (Royal) regular	½ cup	22.0
Lemon:		
(Jell-O) instant	½ cup	31.0
(My-T-Fine) regular	½ cup	30.0

Food and Description	Measure or Quantity	Carbohydrates (grams)
(Royal):		
Regular	½ cup	30.0
Instant	½ cup	29.0
Lime (Royal) regular, Key Lime	½ cup	30.0
Pineapple (Jell-O) instant, cream	½ cup	31.0
Pistachio:		
(Jell-O) instant	½ cup	30.0
(Royal) instant, nut	½ cup	30.0
Rice, *Jell-O Americana*	½ cup	30.0
Tapioca:		
Jell-O Americana, chocolate or vanilla	½ cup	27.0
(My-T-Fine) vanilla	½ cup	28.0
(Royal) vanilla	½ cup	27.0
Vanilla:		
(Jell-O):		
Regular	½ cup	27.0
Regular or instant, French	½ cup	30.0
(My-T-Fine) regular	½ cup	28.0
(Royal):		
Regular	½ cup	27.0
Instant	½ cup	29.0
*Mix, dietetic:		
Butterscotch:		
(D-Zerta)	½ cup	13.0
(Featherweight) artificially sweetened	½ cup	9.0
Chocolate:		
(Dia-Mel)	½ cup	8.2
(Estee)	½ cup	11.0
(Featherweight) artificially sweetened	½ cup	9.0
Lemon:		
(Dia-Mel)	½ cup	8.2
(Estee)	½ cup	26.6
Vanilla:		
(Estee)	½ cup	16.0
(Featherweight) artificially sweetened	½ cup	9.0
PUFFED RICE, cereal:		
(Malt-O-Meal)	½ oz.	12.0
(Quaker)	1 cup	12.7
PUFFED WHEAT, cereal:		
(Malt-O-Meal)	1 cup	11.0
(Quaker)	1 cup	10.8
PUMPKIN, canned:		
(Del Monte)	½ cup	9.5

Food and Description	Measure or Quantity	Carbohydrates (grams)
(Libby's)	4-oz. serving	9.9
(Stokely-Van Camp)	½ cup	9.5
PUMPKIN SEED, in hull	1 oz.	3.2

Q

QUAIL, raw, meat & skin	4 oz.	0.
QUIK (Nestlé):		
Chocolate	1 tsp.	9.5
Strawberry	1 tsp.	11.0
QUINCE JAM (Smucker's)	1 T.	13.5
QUISP, cereal (Quaker)	1⅛ cups	23.1

R

RADISH	2 small radishes	.7
RAISIN, dried:		
(Del Monte)	3 oz.	67.8
(Sun-Maid)	3 oz.	66.0
RAISINS, RICE & RYE, cereal		
(Kellogg's)	¾ cup	31.0
RALSTON, cereal	¼ cup	20.0
RASPBERRY:		
Fresh, trimmed, black	½ cup	10.5
Fresh, trimmed, red	½ cup	9.8
Frozen (Birds Eye) quick thaw	5-oz. serving	34.8
RASPBERRY PRESERVE or JAM:		
Sweetened (Smucker's)	1 T.	13.5
Dietetic:		
(Dia-Mel) black	1 T.	0.
(Featherweight) red	1 T	4.0
(S&W) *Nutradiet*, red	1 T.	3.0
RASPBERRY SPREAD, low sugar		
(Smucker's)	1 T.	6.0
RAVIOLI:		
Canned, regular pack:		
(Franco-American):		
Beef, in meat sauce	7½-oz. can	36.0
Beef, *Raviolios*, in meat sauce	7½-oz. can	32.0
Cheese, in tomato sauce, *Raviolios*	7½-oz. can	39.0
(Nalley's) beef or chicken	8-oz. serving	34.1
Canned, dietetic (Dia-Mel) beef, in sauce	8-oz. can	35.0
RELISH:		
Hamburger (Nalley's)	1 T.	4.1

Food and Description	*Measure or Quantity*	*Carbohydrates (grams)*
Hot dog (Nalley's)	1 T.	4.8
Sour	1 T.	.4
Sweet:		
(Nalley's)	1 T.	3.9
(Smucker's)	1 T.	4.8
RHINE WINE:		
(Great Western)	3 fl. oz.	2.9
(Taylor)	3 fl. oz.	3.0
RHUBARB, cooked, sweetened	½ cup	43.2
***RICE:**		
Brown:		
(River) natural	½ cup	23.0
(Uncle Ben's) parboiled, added butter	⅔ cup	26.4
White:		
(Minute Rice) instant, no added butter	⅔ cup	27.0
(River) medium grain	½ cup	22.0
(Success) long grain	½ cup	23.0
White & wild (Carolina) parboiled	½ cup	20.0
RICE FRIED (See also RICE MIX):		
*Canned (La Choy):	⅓ of 11-oz. can	39.7
Frozen:		
(La Choy) & pork	6-oz. serving	38.8
(Temple) shrimp	1 cup	51.0
***RICE, FRIED, SEASONING MIX** (Durkee)	1 cup	46.5
RICE KRINKLES, cereal (Post)	⅞ cup	26.3
RICE KRISPIES, cereal (Kellogg's)	1 cup	25.0
RICE MIX:		
Beef:		
(Ann Page) *Rice 'n Easy*	⅙ of pkg.	26.2
*(Carolina) *Bake-It-Easy*	⅙ of 6-oz. pkg.	23.0
Rice-A-Roni	⅙ of 8-oz. pkg.	26.0
Chicken:		
(Ann Page) *Rice 'n Easy*	⅙ of pkg.	27.4
*(Carolina) *Bake-It-Easy*	⅙ of 6-oz. pkg.	23.0
Rice-A-Roni	⅙ of pkg.	33.2
*Drumstock (Minute Rice)	½ cup	25.0
*Fried (Minute Rice)	½ cup	25.0
*Long grain & wild (Uncle Ben's) with butter	½ cup	20.6
*Oriental (Carolina) *Bake-It-Easy*	⅙ of pkg.	23.0
*Rib roast (Minute Rice)	½ cup	25.0
Spanish:		
*(Carolina) *Bake-It-Easy*	⅙ of 6-oz. pkg.	23.0
*(Minute Rice)	½ cup	25.0
Rice-A-Roni	⅙ of 7½-oz. pkg.	25.9

Food and Description	Measure or Quantity	Carbohydrates (grams)
RICE, SPANISH, canned:		
(Comstock)	½ of 7½-oz. can	27.0
(Libby's)	7½-oz. serving	27.5
(Menner's)	½ of 7½-oz. can	27.0
(Van Camp)	½ cup	15.5
RICE & VEGETABLES, frozen:		
(Birds Eye) with peas & mushrooms	⅓ of pkg.	22.4
(Green Giant):		
& broccoli in cheese sauce	½ of 11-oz. pkg.	22.7
Continental, with green bean & almonds	½ of 11-oz. pkg.	21.4
Medley, with peas and mushrooms	½ of 11-oz. pkg.	23.7
Pilaf, with mushrooms and onions	½ of 11-oz. pkg.	28.7
Verdi, with bell pepper and parsley	½ of 11-oz. pkg.	32.0
RICE WINE:		
Chinese, 20.7% alcohol	1 fl. oz.	1.1
Japanese, 10.6% alcohol	1 fl. oz.	12.1
Non-alcoholic	1 oz.	6.6
RIESLING WINE, Grey (Inglenook)	3 fl. oz.	.7
ROAST BEEF SPREAD		
(Underwood)	1-oz. serving	.3
ROCKFISH, steamed	4-oz. serving	2.2
ROCK & RYE (Mr. Boston)	1 fl. oz.	7.2
ROE, baked or broiled, cod & shad	4-oz. serving	2.2
ROLAIDS	1 piece	1.4
ROLL or BUN:		
Regular, not frozen:		
Biscuit (Wonder)	1 roll	17.1
Brown & serve (Wonder) *Gem Style*	1 roll	13.6
Club (Pepperidge Farm)	1 roll	20.0
Crescent (Pepperidge Farm) butter	1 roll	13.0
Deli twist (Arnold)	1 roll	17.0
Dinner:		
Home Pride	1-oz. roll	13.6
(Pepperidge Farm)	1 roll	10.0
(Wonder)	1¼-oz. roll	17.0
Dinner Party Rounds (Arnold)	.7-oz. roll	10.0
Finger:		
(Arnold) *Dinner Party*	1 roll	10.0
(Pepperidge Farm):		
Poppy	1 roll	8.0
Sesame	1 roll	8.7

Food and Description	Measure or Quantity	Carbohydrates (grams)
Frankfurter:		
(Arnold) hot dog	1 roll	20.0
(Wonder)	2-oz. roll	28.9
French:		
(Arnold) *Francisco, Sourdough*	1.1-oz. roll	16.0
(Pepperidge Farm):		
Small	1 roll	48.0
Large	1 roll	76.0
Golden Twist (Pepperidge Farm)	1 roll	14.0
Hamburger:		
(Arnold)	1 roll	21.0
(Pepperidge Farm)	1 roll	18.0
Roman Meal	1 roll	36.1
(Wonder)	2-oz. roll	29.1
Hearth (Pepperidge Farm)	1 roll	10.0
Honey (Hostess)	1 cake	63.4
Kaiser-Hogie (Wonder)	6-oz. roll	81.8
Old fashioned (Pepperidge Farm)	1 roll	7.7
Parkerhouse:		
(Arnold) *Dinner Party*	1 roll	10.0
(Pepperidge Farm)	1 roll	9.0
Party pan (Pepperidge Farm)	1 roll	5.3
Sandwich (Arnold) soft	1 roll	18.0
Sesame crisp (Pepperidge Farm)	1 roll	11.0
Frozen:		
Apple crunch (Sara Lee)	1-oz. roll	13.5
Caramel pecan (Sara Lee)	1.3-oz. roll	17.4
Caramel sticky (Sara Lee)	1 bun	15.2
Cinnamon (Sara Lee)	.9-oz. roll	13.9
Croissants (Sara Lee)	.9-oz. roll	11.2
Crumb (Sara Lee):		
Blueberry	1¾-oz. bun	26.8
French	1.7-oz. bun	29.9
Danish (Sara Lee):		
Apple	1.3-oz. roll	17.4
Apple country	1.8-oz. roll	22.9
Cheese	1.3-oz. roll	13.9
Cheese country	1½-oz. roll	13.5
Cherry	1.3-oz. roll	16.4
Cherry country	1.6-oz. roll	18.9
Cinnamon raisin	1.3-oz. roll	17.3
Pecan	1.3-oz. roll	18.3
Honey:		
(Morton):		
Regular	2¼-oz. roll	30.7

Food and Description	Measure or Quantity	Carbohydrates (grams)
Mini	1.3-oz. roll	17.7
(Sara Lee)	1-oz. roll	15.2
*ROLL DOUGH:		
Frozen (Richs'):		
Cinnamon	1 roll	32.8
Frankfurter	1 roll	24.9
Onion, regular	1 roll	29.1
Refrigerated (Pillsbury):		
Caramel danish with nuts	1 roll	19.5
Cinnamon with icing	1 roll	17.5
Cinnamon with icing, *Ballard*	1 roll	17.0
Cinnamon with icing, *Hungry Jack, Butter Tastin*	1 roll	19.5
Cinnamon raisin danish	1 roll	20.0
Crescent, *Ballard*	1 roll	26.0
Orange danish	1 roll	19.5
Wheat, bakery style	1 roll	16.0
White, bakery style	1 roll	18.0
*ROLL MIX, hot (Pillsbury)	1 roll	15.5
ROMAN MEAL, cereal	⅓ cup	20.0
ROSEMARY LEAVES (French's)	1 tsp.	.8
ROSÉ WINE:		
(Great Western)	3 fl. oz.	2.4
(Mogen David)	3 fl. oz.	8.9
(Paul Masson):		
Regular, 11.8% alcohol	3 fl. oz.	4.2
Light, 7.1% alcohol	3 fl. oz.	3.9
ROTINI IN TOMATO SAUCE, canned (Franco-American):		
Plain	7½-oz. can	36.0
& meatball	7⅜-oz. can	29.0
RUTABAGA:		
Canned (Sunshine) solids & liq.	½ cup	6.9
Frozen (Southland)	4 oz.	13.0

S

SAFFLOWER SEED, in hull	1 oz.	1.8
SAGE (French's)	1 tsp.	.6
SAINT-EMILION (B&G)	3 fl. oz.	.7
SAKÉ WINE	1 fl. oz.	1.4
SALAD DRESSING:		
Regular:		
Avocado Goddess (Marie's)	1 T.	1.0
Bacon (Seven Seas) creamy	1 T.	1.0
Bell pepper (Seven Seas) *Viva*	1 T.	1.0

Food and Description	Measure or Quantity	Carbohydrates (grams)
Bleu or blue cheese:		
(Bernstein) Danish	1 T.	.6
(Seven Seas) chunky	1 T.	1.0
(Wish-Bone) chunky	1 T.	1.0
Caesar:		
(Pfeiffer)	1 T.	.5
(Seven Seas) *Viva*	1 T.	1.0
(Wish-Bone)	1 T.	1.0
Capri (Seven Seas)	1 T.	3.0
Cucumber (Wish-Bone) creamy	1 T.	2.0
French:		
(Bernstein's) creamy	1 T.	2.1
(Nalley's)	1 T.	2.1
(Pfeiffer)	1 T.	3.5
(Seven Seas) creamy	1 T.	2.0
(Wish-Bone) deluxe	1 T.	3.0
Garlic (Wish-Bone) creamy	1 T.	2.0
Green Goddess:		
(Seven Seas)	1 T.	0.
(Wish-Bone)	1 T.	1.0
Herb & spice (Seven Seas)	1 T.	1.0
Italian:		
(Bernstein's)	1 T.	.8
(Marie's)	1 T.	1.1
(Pfeiffer) chef	1 T.	.5
(Seven Seas)	1 T.	1.0
(Wish-Bone)	1 T.	1.0
Louis Dressing (Nalley's)	1 T.	1.8
Onion 'N Chive (Seven Seas) creamy	1 T.	1.0
Ranch (Marie's)	1 T.	1.3
Red wine vinegar & oil (Seven Seas)	1 T.	1.0
Roquefort:		
(Bernstein's)	1 T.	.8
(Marie's)	1 T.	1.1
Russian:		
(Pfeiffer)	1 T.	2.0
(Seven Seas) creamy	1 T.	1.0
Spin Blend (Hellmann's)	1 T.	2.7
Sweet 'N Sour (Dutch Pantry) creamy	1 T.	4.0
Thousand Island:		
(Marie's)	1 T.	1.6
(Pfeiffer)	1 T.	2.0
(Seven Seas)	1 T.	2.0
Vinaigrette (Bernstein's) French	1 T.	.2

Food and Description	Measure or Quantity	Carbohydrates (grams)
Dietetic:		
Bleu or blue cheese:		
(Featherweight)	1 T.	1.0
(Tillie Lewis) *Tasti-Diet*	1 T.	<1.0
(Walden Farms) chunky	1 T.	1.5
Caesar:		
(Estee)	1 T.	1.0
(Pfeiffer)	1 T.	1.0
Cucumber (Wish-Bone) creamy	1 T.	1.0
Cucumber & onion (Feather-weight) creamy	1 T.	1.0
French:		
(Featherweight) imitation	1 T.	1.0
(Pfeiffer)	1 T.	2.5
(Tillie Lewis) *Tasti-Diet*	1 T.	<1.0
(Walden Farms) chunky	1 T.	3.0
(Wish-Bone)	1 T.	4.0
Herb & Spice (Featherweight)	1 T.	1.0
Imitation (Featherweight)	1 T.	1.0
Italian:		
(Estee) spicy	1 T.	1.0
(Featherweight)	1 T.	1.0
(Pfeiffer)	1 T.	1.5
(Tillie Lewis) *Tasti-Diet*	1 T.	Tr.
(Walden Farms) *classico*	1 T.	1.5
(Weight Watchers)	1 T.	2.0
(Wish-Bone)	1 T.	1.0
Red wine (Pfeiffer)	1 T.	1.0
Red wine/vinegar (Feather-weight)	1 T.	1.0
Russian:		
(Dia-Mel)	1 T.	.5
(Featherweight) creamy	1 T.	1.0
(Pfeiffer)	1 T.	2.0
(Tillie Lewis) *Tasti-Diet*	1 T.	<1.0
(Weight Watchers)	1 T.	2.0
(Wish-Bone)	1 T.	5.0
Thousand Island:		
(Featherweight)	1 T.	1.1
(Pfeiffer)	1 T.	2.0
(Walden Farms)	1 T.	3.0
(Weight Watchers)	1 T.	2.0
(Wish-Bone)	1 T.	3.0
2-Calorie Low Sodium (Feather-weight)	1 T.	0.
Whipped:		
(Dia-Mel)	1 T.	2.1
(Tillie Lewis) *Tasti-Diet*	1 T.	1.0

Food and Description	Measure or Quantity	Carbohydrates (grams)
SALAD DRESSING MIX:		
*Regular (Good Seasons):		
Bleu or blue cheese:		
Regular	1 T.	.5
Thick'n Creamy	1 T.	.5
Buttermilk Farm Style	1 T.	1.0
French:		
Old fashioned	1 T.	1.0
Thick'n Creamy	1 T.	2.0
Garlic	1 T.	1.0
Italian	1 T.	1.0
Onion	1 T.	1.0
Thousand Island, *Thick'n Creamy*	1 T.	2.0
Dietetic:		
*Bleu cheese (Weight Watchers)	1 T.	1.0
French:		
(Dia-Mel)	½-oz. packet	0.
*(Weight Watchers)	1 T.	1.0
Garlic (Dia-Mel) creamy	½-oz. packet	1.0
Italian:		
(Dia-Mel)	½-oz. packet	0.
*(Good Seasons)	1 T.	2.0
*(Weight Watchers) regular	1 T.	0.
*(Weight Watchers) creamy	1 T.	1.0
Russian:		
(Louis Sherry)	½-oz. packet	0.
*(Weight Watchers)	1 T.	1.0
Thousand Island:		
(Dia-Mel)	½-oz. packet	0.
*(Weight Watchers)	1 T.	1.0
SALAD FIXIN'S (Arnold):		
Danish-style blue cheese or French onion	½ oz.	8.8
Spicy Italian	½ oz.	8.7
SALAD LIFT SPICE (French's)	1 tsp.	1.0
SALAD SEASONING (Durkee):		
Regular	1 tsp.	.7
With cheese	1 tsp.	.4
SALAMI:		
(Hormel):		
Cotto	1-oz. slice	0.
Genoa, *Di Lusso*	1-oz. serving	< .1
Genoa, sliced	1-oz. serving	.6
Hard, sliced	1-oz. serving	.4
(Oscar Mayer):		
For beer, beef	.8-oz. slice	.2

117

Food and Description	Measure or Quantity	Carbohydrate (grams)
Cotto	½-oz. slice	.2
Cotto, beef	.8-oz. slice	.6
Hard	.3-oz. slice	.2
(Oscherwitz) sliced	1-oz. serving	.9
(Swift)	1-oz. serving	.3
(Vienna) beef	1-oz. serving	.8
SALISBURY STEAK:		
Canned (Morton House)	½ of 12½-oz. can	7.0
Frozen:		
(Banquet):		
Buffet Supper	2-lb. pkg.	48.2
Man-Pleaser	19-oz. dinner	71.7
(Green Giant) with gravy, oven bake	7-oz. serving	14.0
(Morton) *Country Table*	12-oz. dinner	60.0
(Stouffer's) with onion gravy	6-oz. serving	4.9
(Swanson):		
With gravy	10-oz. entree	16.0
Hungry Man	17-oz. dinner	63.0
3-course	16-oz. dinner	47.0
TV Brand	11½-oz. dinner	40.0
SALMON:		
Baked or broiled	6¾″ x 2½″ x 1″	0.
Canned	Any quantity	0.
SALMON, SMOKED (Vita):		
Lox, drained	4-oz. jar	.2
Nova, drained	4-oz. can	1.0
SALT:		
Regular (Morton):		
Lite Salt	1 tsp.	0.
Table	1 tsp.	0.
Substitute:		
(Adolph's):		
Plain	1 tsp.	Tr.
Seasoned	1 tsp.	1.1
(Morton) plain	1 tsp.	Tr.
Salt-It (Dia-Mel)	1 tsp.	0.
SANDWICH SPREAD:		
(Hellmann's)	1 T.	2.3
(Nalley's)	1 T.	3.0
(Oscar Mayer)	1-oz. serving	3.2
SANGRIA (Taylor)	3 fl. oz.	10.8
SARDINE, canned:		
Atlantic (Del Monte) with tomato sauce	7½-oz. can	4.0
Imported (Underwood) in tomato or mustard sauce	3¾-oz. can	1.0

118

Food and Description	Measure or Quantity	Carbohydrates (grams)
Norwegian, *King Oscar Brand:*		
In mustard or tomato sauce	3¾-oz. can	2.0
In oil, drained	3-oz. can	1.0
SAUCE:		
A.1.	1 T.	3.1
Barbecue:		
Chris & Pitt's	1 T.	4.0
(French's)	1 T.	3.0
(Gold's)	1 T.	3.9
Open Pit (General Foods) hickory smoke	1 T.	4.0
Cocktail:		
(Gold's)	1-oz. serving	7.5
(Nalley's)	1-oz. serving	7.1
(Pfeiffer)	1-oz. serving	12.0
Escoffier Sauce Diable	1 T.	4.3
Escoffier Sauce Robert	1 T.	5.1
Famous Sauce	1 T.	2.2
Hot, *Frank's*	1 tsp.	0.
H.P. Steak Sauce	1 T.	4.8
Italian:		
(Carnation)	2 fl. oz.	7.0
(Ragu) red cooking	3½ oz.	6.0
Marinara (Ragu)	5-oz. serving	15.0
Mushroom (Nalley's)	1-oz. serving	2.0
Salsa Picante (Del Monte)	¼ cup	3.0
Salsa Roja (Del Monte)	¼ cup	4.0
Seafood (Bernstein's)	1 T.	3.6
Seafood cocktail (Del Monte)	1 T.	4.9
Soy:		
(Gold's)	1 T.	1.0
(Kikkoman)	1 T.	1.1
(La Choy)	1 T.	.9
Spare rib (Gold's)	1 T.	11.7
Steak (Dawn Fresh) with mushrooms	2-oz. serving	3.5
Steak Supreme	1 T.	5.1
Sweet & sour:		
(Carnation)	2 fl. oz.	16.0
(La Choy)	1 oz.	12.6
Swiss steak (Carnation)	2-oz. serving	4.5
Taco:		
(Del Monte) hot or mild	¼ cup	4.0
Old El Paso	1-oz. serving	2.3
(Ortega)	1 T.	5.1
Tartar:		
(Hellmann's)	1 T.	.2

Food and Description	Measure or Quantity	Carbohydrates (grams)
(Nalley's)	1 T.	.3
Teriyaki (Kikkoman)	1 T.	2.8
V-8	1-oz. serving	6.0
White, medium	¼ cup	5.6
Worcestershire:		
(French's)	1 T.	2.0
(Gold's)	1 T.	3.3
SAUCE MIX:		
Regular:		
A la King (Durkee)	1.1-oz. pkg.	14.0
*Cheese:		
(Durkee)	¼ cup	4.8
(French's)	¼ cup	7.0
Hollandaise:		
(Durkee)	1-oz. pkg.	11.0
*(French's)	1 T.	.7
*Sour cream:		
(Durkee)	⅔ cup	15.0
(French's)	2½ T.	5.0
*Stroganoff (French's)	⅓ cup	11.0
*Sweet and sour:		
(Durkee)	¼ cup	11.2
(French's)	¼ cup	7.0
*Teriyaki (French's)	1 T.	3.5
*White (Durkee)	½ cup	20.5
*Dietetic (Weight Watchers) lemon butter	1 T.	1.0
SAUERKRAUT, canned:		
(Claussen) drained	½ cup	2.8
(Del Monte) solids & liq.	½ cup	5.3
(Libby's) solids & liq.	4-oz. serving	4.8
(Silver Floss) solids & liq.:		
Regular	½ cup	5.0
Bavarian kraut	½ cup	8.0
(Stokely-Van Camp) Bavarian style, solids & liq.	½ cup	7.0
SAUSAGE:		
*Brown 'N Serve (Swift) original	.8-oz. link	.5
Italian-style (Best's Kosher; Oscherwitz)	3-oz. link	.7
Polish-style:		
(Best's Kosher; Oscherwitz)	3-oz. link	1.8
(Vienna)	3-oz. link	1.3
Pork:		
*(Hormel) *Little Sizzlers*	1 link	Tr.
(Jimmy Dean)	2-oz. serving	Tr.
(Oscar Mayer) *Little Friers*	.6-oz. link	.4

Food and Description	Measure or Quantity	Carbohydrates (grams)
Smoked:		
(Best's Kosher; Oscherwitz)	3-oz. link	2.4
(Eckrich) beef, *Smok-Y-Links*	.8-oz. link	1.0
(Hormel) pork	3-oz. serving	.7
(Oscar Mayer)	1½-oz. link	.6
(Vienna)	2½-oz. serving	.9
*Turkey (Louis Rich) links or tube	1-oz. serving	<1.0
SAUTERNE WINE:		
(Great Western)	3 fl. oz.	4.5
(Taylor)	3 fl. oz.	4.8
SAVORY (French's)	1 tsp.	1.0
SCALLOP:		
Fresh, steamed	4-oz. serving	DNA
Frozen:		
(Mrs. Paul's):		
Breaded & fried	½ of 7-oz. pkg.	24.1
With butter & cheese	7-oz. pkg.	11.2
(Van de Kamp's) country seasoned	½ of 7-oz. pkg.	19.0
SCHAV SOUP, canned (Gold's)	8-oz. serving	2.1
SCHNAPPS, PEPPERMINT (Mr. Boston)	1 fl. oz.	8.0
*SCOTCH BROTH SOUP, canned (Campbell)	10-oz. serving	11.0
SCREWDRIVER COCKTAIL, canned (Mr. Boston) 12½% alcohol	3 fl. oz.	12.0
SEAFOOD PLATTER, frozen (Mrs. Paul's) breaded and fried	½ of 9-oz. pkg.	28.5
SEAFOOD SEASONING (French's)	1 tsp.	Tr.
SEGO DIET FOOD:		
Bars	1 bar	12.0
Canned:		
Milk chocolate, very chocolate and very chocolate coconut	10-fl.-oz. can	39.0
Very banana, very vanilla	10-fl.-oz. can	34.0
SERUTAN:		
Toasted granules	1 tsp.	1.3
Concentrated powder	1 tsp.	1.3
Fruit-flavored powder	1 tsp.	1.5
SESAME SEEDS (French's)	1 tsp.	.9
SHAD, CREOLE	4-oz. serving	1.9
SHAKE 'N BAKE:		
Regular:		
Chicken	2.4-oz. pkg.	43.0
Chicken, barbecue style	3¾-oz. pkg.	83.2
Chicken, crispy country milk	2.3-oz. pkg.	50.1
Chicken, Italian flavor	2.3-oz. pkg.	41.4

Food and Description	Measure or Quantity	Carbohydrates (grams)
Fish	2-oz. pkg.	33.9
Hamburger	2-oz. pkg.	33.2
Pork	2.4-oz. pkg.	47.1
Pork & ribs, barbecue style	2.9-oz. pkg.	61.2
Plus home-style gravy mix:		
Beef	3.2-oz. pkg.	51.4
Pork	3.7-oz. pkg.	67.4
SHERBET:		
(Baskin-Robbins) Daiquiri Ice or orange	1 scoop	20.9
(Meadow Gold) orange	¼ pint	26.0
SHERRY:		
Cocktail (Gold Seal)	3 fl. oz.	1.6
Cream:		
(Great Western) Solera	3 fl. oz.	12.2
(Taylor)	3 fl. oz.	13.2
Dry:		
(Italian Swiss Colony) *Gold Medal*	3 fl. oz.	1.7
(Williams & Humbert)	3 fl. oz.	4.5
Dry Sack (Williams & Humbert)	3 fl. oz.	4.5
SHREDDED WHEAT:		
(Nabisco):		
Regular	¾-oz. biscuit	23.0
Spoon Size	⅔ cup	23.0
(Quaker)	1 biscuit	11.0
SHRIMP:		
Canned:		
(Bumble Bee) solids & liq.	4½-oz. can	.9
(Icy Point) cocktail	4½-oz. can	.8
Frozen (Mrs. Paul's) fried	½ of 6-oz. pkg.	16.8
SHRIMP CAKE, frozen (Mrs. Paul's) thins	2½-oz. cake	1.4
SHRIMP DINNER, frozen (Van de Kamp's)	10-oz. dinner	40.0
SHRIMP PUFF, frozen (Durkee)	1 piece	3.0
SHRIMP SOUP:		
*(Campbell) cream of:		
Made with milk	10-oz. serving	17.0
Made with water	10-oz. serving	10.0
(Crosse & Blackwell)	6½-oz. serving	7.0
SHRIMP STICKS, frozen (Mrs. Paul's)	.8-oz. stick	5.5
SIRLOIN BURGER SOUP		
(Campbell) *Chunky*	10½-oz. can	23.0
SLENDER (Carnation):		
Bar	1 bar	11.5

Food and Description	Measure or Quantity	Carbohydrates (grams)
Dry	1 packet	20.0
Liquid	10-fl.-oz. can	34.0
SLIM JIM	1 piece	.4
SLOPPY HOT DOG SEASONING		
MIX (French's)	1½-oz. pkg.	28.0
SLOPPY JOE:		
Canned:		
(Hormel) *Short Orders*	7½-oz. can	15.0
(Libby's):		
Beef	⅓ cup	6.0
Pork	⅓ cup	5.7
(Morton House) beef	5-oz. serving	19.0
(Nalley's)	8-oz. serving	25.0
Frozen:		
(Banquet) *Cookin' Bag*	5-oz. bag	11.2
(Green Giant) with tomato sauce & beef, *Toast Topper*	5-oz. serving	14.3
SLOPPY JOE SEASONING MIX:		
*(Durkee):		
Regular	1¼ cups	30.0
Pizza flavor	1¼ cups	26.0
(French's)	1½-oz. pkg.	32.0
SNO BALL (Hostess)	1 cake	25.1
SOAVE WINE (Antinori)	3 fl. oz.	6.3
SOFT DRINK:		
Sweetened:		
Apple (Welch's)	6 fl. oz.	23.5
Aspen	6 fl. oz.	18.6
Bitter lemon:		
(Canada Dry)	6 fl. oz.	19.2
(Schweppes)	6 fl. oz.	20.3
Bubble Up	6 fl. oz.	18.4
Cherry:		
(Canada Dry) wild	6 fl. oz.	24.0
(Shasta) black	6 fl. oz.	21.5
Chocolate (Yoo-Hoo) high protein	6 fl. oz.	24.1
Club (all brands)	6 fl. oz.	0.
Coconut (Yoo-Hoo)	6 fl. oz.	18.0
Cola:		
(Canada Dry) *Jamaica*	6 fl. oz.	19.8
Coca-Cola	6 fl. oz.	18.0
Pepsi-Cola	6 fl. oz.	19.8
(Royal Crown)	6 fl. oz.	19.4
(Shasta):		
Regular	6 fl. oz.	19.5
Cherry	6 fl. oz.	18.5

Food and Description	Measure or Quantity	Carbohydrates (grams)
Cream:		
(Canada Dry) vanilla	6 fl. oz.	24.0
(Schweppes) red	6 fl. oz.	21.3
(Shasta)	6 fl. oz.	20.5
Dr. Nehi (Royal Crown)	6 fl. oz.	18.3
Dr. Pepper	6 fl. oz.	19.4
Fruit punch:		
(Nehi)	6 fl. oz.	22.8
(Shasta)	6 fl. oz.	23.0
Ginger ale:		
(Canada Dry)	6 fl. oz.	15.6
(Fanta)	6 fl. oz.	15.8
(Nehi)	6 fl. oz.	16.6
(Schweppes)	6 fl. oz.	16.3
(Shasta)	6 fl. oz.	16.0
Ginger beer (Schweppes)	6 fl.oz.	16.8
Grape:		
(Canada Dry) concord	6 fl. oz.	24.0
(Fanta)	6 fl. oz.	21.8
(Hi-C)	6 fl. oz.	20.0
(Nehi)	6 fl. oz.	21.8
(Patio)	6 fl. oz.	24.0
(Schweppes)	6 fl. oz.	15.7
(Shasta)	6 fl. oz.	23.5
(Welch's) sparkling	6 fl. oz.	23.0
Hi Spot (Canada Dry)	6 fl. oz.	18.6
Kick (Royal Crown)	6 fl. oz.	22.1
Lemonade (Shasta)	6 fl. oz.	19.0
Lemon-lime (Shasta)	6 fl. oz.	19.0
Mello Yello	6 fl. oz.	22.5
Mountain Dew	6 fl. oz.	22.2
Mr. PiBB	6 fl. oz.	18.8
Orange:		
(Canada Dry) *Sunripe*	6 fl. oz.	14.1
(Fanta)	6 fl. oz.	22.5
(Hi-C)	6 fl. oz.	20.0
(Nehi)	6 fl. oz.	23.8
(Patio)	6 fl. oz.	24.0
(Schweppes) sparkling	6 fl. oz.	22.0
(Shasta)	6 fl. oz.	23.5
(Sunkist)	6 fl. oz.	7.6
(Welch's)	6 fl. oz.	23.5
Peach (Nehi)	6 fl. oz.	23.0
Quinine or Tonic Water:		
(Canada Dry)	6 fl. oz.	16.1
(Schweppes)	6 fl. oz.	16.5
(Shasta)	6 fl. oz.	16.0
Rondo (Schweppes)	6 fl. oz.	19.6

Food and Description	Measure or Quantity	Carbohydrates (grams)
Root Beer:		
Barrelhead (Canada Dry)	6 fl. oz.	19.8
(Dad's)	6 fl. oz.	19.6
(Fanta)	6 fl. oz.	20.3
(Nehi)	6 fl. oz.	21.8
On Tap	6 fl. oz.	20.4
(Patio)	6 fl. oz.	21.0
Rooti (Canada Dry)	6 fl. oz.	19.8
(Shasta) draft	6 fl. oz.	20.5
Seven-Up	6 fl. oz.	18.1
Sprite	6 fl. oz.	18.0
Strawberry:		
(Canada Dry) California	6 fl. oz.	22.3
(Nehi)	6 fl. oz.	21.8
(Shasta)	6 fl. oz.	19.5
(Welch's)	6 fl. oz.	23.5
(Yoo-Hoo)	6 fl. oz.	20.9
Tahitian Treat (Canada Dry)	6 fl. oz.	24.1
Teem	6 fl. oz.	18.6
Tom Collins or Collins Mix		
(Canada Dry)	6 fl. oz.	15.0
Upper 10 (Royal Crown)	6 fl. oz.	19.0
Vanilla:		
(Canada Dry) cream	6 fl. oz.	22.0
(Yoo-Hoo) shake	6 fl. oz.	20.4
Wink (Canada Dry)	6 fl. oz.	22.7
Dietetic or low calorie:		
Bubble Up	6 fl. oz.	.2
Cherry:		
(Shasta) black	6 fl. oz.	Tr.
(Tab) black	6 fl. oz.	Tr.
Chocolate (No-Cal) mint	6 fl. oz.	Tr.
Cola:		
(Canada Dry)	6 fl. oz.	.6
Diet Rite	6 fl. oz.	Tr.
(No-Cal)	6 fl. oz.	Tr.
Pepsi, diet	6 fl. oz.	Tr.
Pepsi Light	6 fl. oz.	Tr.
RC	6 fl. oz.	Tr.
(Shasta) regular or cherry	6 fl. oz.	Tr.
Tab	6 fl. oz.	Tr.
Cream:		
(No-Cal)	6 fl. oz.	Tr.
(Shasta)	6 fl. oz.	Tr.
Dr. Pepper	6 fl. oz	.4
Fresca	6 fl. oz.	0.
Ginger ale:		
(Canada Dry)	6 fl. oz.	0.

Food and Description	Measure or Quantity	Carbohydrates (grams)
(No-Cal)	6 fl. oz.	Tr.
(Shasta)	6 fl. oz.	Tr.
Tab	6 fl. oz.	Tr.
Grape:		
(Shasta)	6 fl. oz.	Tr.
Tab	6 fl. oz.	0.
Grapefruit (Shasta)	6 fl. oz.	.2
Lemon-lime:		
(Shasta)	6 fl. oz.	Tr.
Tab	6 fl. oz.	0.
Mr. PiBB	6 fl. oz.	0.
Orange:		
(No-Cal)	6 fl. oz.	0.
Tab	6 fl. oz.	0.
Red Pop (No-Cal)	6 fl. oz.	0.
Rondo (Schweppes)	6 fl. oz.	Tr.
Root Beer:		
Barrelhead (Canada Dry)	6 fl. oz.	.8
(Dad's)	6 fl. oz.	.2
(No-Cal)	6 fl. oz.	Tr.
(Shasta) draft	6 fl. oz.	Tr.
Tab	6 fl. oz.	Tr.
Seven-Up	6 fl. oz.	0.
Shape-Up (No-Cal)	6 fl. oz.	0.
Sprite	6 fl. oz.	0.
Strawberry (Shasta)	6 fl. oz.	Tr.
Tab	6 fl. oz.	0.
SOLE, frozen:		
(Mrs. Paul's):		
Fillets, breaded and fried	4-oz. serving	21.8
Fillets, with lemon butter	4½-oz. serving	9.7
(Van de Kamp's) batter dipped, french fried	1 piece	12.0
(Weight Watchers) in lemon sauce	9¼-oz. meal	17.0
SOUFFLÉ, frozen (Stouffer's) cheese	6-oz. serving	13.9
SOUP GREENS (Durkee)	2½-oz. can	43.0
SOUTHERN COMFORT, 86 or 100 proof	1 fl. oz.	3.5
SOYBEAN CURD or TOFU	2¾" x 1½" x 1" cake	2.9
SOYBEAN or NUT:		
Dry roasted (Soy Ahoy; Soy Town)	1 oz.	6.0
Oil roasted (Soy Ahoy; Soy Town) plain, barbecue or garlic flavor	1 oz.	4.8
SPAGHETTI:		
Cooked:		
8-10 minutes, "al dente"	1 cup	43.9

Food and Description	Measure or Quantity	Carbohydrates (grams)
14-20 minutes, tender	1 cup	32.2
Canned:		
(Franco-American):		
With little meatballs in tomato sauce, *SpaghettiOs*	7⅜-oz. can	24.0
With meatballs in tomato sauce	7⅜-oz. can	26.0
In meat sauce	7½-oz. can	26.0
With sliced franks in tomato sauce, *SpaghettiOs*	7⅜-oz. can	26.0
In tomato sauce with cheese	7⅜-oz. can	33.0
(Hormel) *Short Orders,* & meatballs in tomato sauce	7½-oz. can	24.0
(Libby's) & meatballs in tomato sauce	7½-oz. can	27.5
(Nally's) & meatballs	8-oz. serving	31.8
Frozen:		
(Banquet):		
Buffet Supper, & meatballs	2-lb. pkg.	129.1
Dinner, & meatballs	11½-oz. pkg.	62.9
(Green Giant) & meatballs in tomato sauce	9-oz. entree	29.1
(Morton) & meatballs	11-oz. dinner	59.4
(Stouffer's) & meat sauce	14-oz. pkg.	61.6
(Swanson) & meatballs, *TV Brand*	12½-oz. dinner	57.0
SPAGHETTI SAUCE:		
Canned, regular pack:		
Clam (Ragu)	5-oz. serving	14.0
Marinara:		
(Prince)	4-oz. serving	12.4
(Ragu)	5-oz. serving	15.0
Meat:		
(Prince)	½ cup	11.0
(Ragu) thick & zesty	5-oz. serving	14.0
(Ronzoni)	4-oz. serving	11.0
Meatless or Plain:		
(Hain)	4-oz. serving	14.2
(Prince)	½ cup	11.4
(Ragu) extra thick & zesty	5-oz. serving	13.0
Mushroom:		
(Hain)	4-oz. serving	14.3
(Prince)	4-oz. serving	11.3
(Ragu)	5-oz. serving	13.0
Pepperoni (Ragu)	5-oz. serving	14.0
Canned, dietetic pack (Featherweight) low sodium	5-oz. serving	10.0

Food and Description	Measure or Quantity	Carbohydrates (grams)
*SPAGHETTI SAUCE MIX:		
(Durkee):		
Plain	½ cup	10.4
Mushroom	1⅓ cups	24.0
(French's)		
Italian style	⅝ cup	15.0
With mushroom	⅝ cup	13.0
(Spatini)	2-oz. serving	4.0
SPAM, luncheon meat (Hormel):		
Regular	1-oz. serving	1.1
& cheese chunks	1-oz. serving	.7
Deviled	1 T.	0.
Smoke flavored	1-oz. serving	.3
SPECIAL K, cereal (Kellogg's)	1 cup	21.0
SPINACH:		
Fresh, whole leaves	½ cup	.7
Fresh, boiled	½ cup	2.8
Canned, regular pack, solids & liq.:		
(Del Monte)	½ cup	3.4
(Sunshine)	½ cup	2.9
Canned, dietetic pack (Feather- weight) low sodium	½ cup	4.0
Frozen:		
(Birds Eye):		
Chopped or leaf	⅓ of pkg.	2.7
Creamed	⅓ of pkg.	4.0
(Green Giant):		
In butter sauce	⅓ of pkg.	2.3
Creamed	⅓ of pkg.	7.8
Soufflé	⅓ of pkg.	8.2
(McKenzie)	⅓ of pkg.	3.3
(Seabrook Farms)	⅓ of pkg.	3.3
(Stouffer's) soufflé	⅓ of pkg.	11.9
SQUASH, SUMMER:		
Yellow, boiled slices	½ cup	2.7
Zucchini, boiled slices	½ cup	1.9
Canned (Del Monte) zucchini in tomato sauce	½ cup	7.9
Frozen:		
(McKenzie) Crookneck	⅓ of pkg.	3.8
(Seabrook Farms):		
Crookneck	⅓ of pkg.	3.8
Zucchini	3½-oz. serving	3.6
(Southland) zucchini, sliced	⅕ of 16-oz. pkg.	3.3
SQUASH, WINTER:		
Acorn, baked	½ cup	14.3
Hubbard, baked, mashed	½ cup	11.9

128

Food and Description	Measure or Quantity	Carbohydrates (grams)
Frozen:		
(Birds Eye)	⅓ of pkg.	11.0
(Southland) butternut	4 oz.	16.0
*START	½ cup	12.7
STEAK & GREEN PEPPERS, frozen (Swanson)	8½-oz. entree	11.0
STEAK & POTATO SOUP (Campbell) *Chunky*	10¾-oz. can	23.0
STOCK BASE (French's)		
Beef	1 tsp.	2.0
Chicken	1 tsp.	1.0
*STOCKPOT SOUP, canned (Campbell) vegetable & beef	11-oz. serving	12.0
STRAWBERRY:		
Fresh, capped	½ cup	6.1
Frozen (Birds Eye):		
Halves	⅓ of pkg.	48.2
Whole	¼ of pkg.	23.2
Whole, quick thaw	½ pkg.	29.7
STRAWBERRY DRINK (Hi-C):		
Canned	6 fl. oz.	22.0
*Mix	6 fl. oz.	17.0
STRAWBERRY ICE CREAM:		
(Baskin-Robbins)	1 scoop (2½ fl. oz.)	15.6
Good Humor	4 fl. oz.	15.0
(Meadow Gold)	¼ pt.	19.0
(Swift)	½ cup	15.3
STRAWBERRY JELLY:		
Sweetened (Smucker's)	1 T.	13.4
Dietetic (Featherweight)	1 T.	4.0
STRAWBERRY PRESERVE or JAM:		
Sweetened:		
(Smucker's)	1 T.	13.5
(Welch's)	1 T.	13.5
Dietetic (See STRAWBERRY SPREAD)		
STRAWBERRY SPREAD, dietetic:		
(Diet Delight)	1 T.	3.0
(Estee)	1 T.	4.8
(Featherweight):		
Regular	1 T.	4.0
Artificially sweetened	1 T.	1.0
(Slenderella)	1 T.	6.0
(S&W) *Nutradiet*	1 T.	3.0
(Tillie Lewis) *Tasti-Diet*	1 T.	3.0
(Welch's) lite	1 T.	6.2
STUFFING MIX:		
*Chicken, *Stove Top*	½ cup	20.0

Food and Description	Measure or Quantity	Carbohydrates (grams)
Cornbread:		
(Pepperidge Farm)	⅛ of 8-oz. pkg.	21.0
*Stove Top	½ cup	20.0
Herb Seasoned (Pepperidge Farm)	⅛ of 8-oz. pkg.	21.0
*Pork, Stove Top	½ cup	20.0
*With rice, Stove Top	½ cup	23.0
White bread, Mrs. Cubbison's	1 oz.	20.5
STURGEON, smoked	4-oz. serving	0.
SUCCOTASH:		
Canned:		
(Libby's) cream style	½ cup	22.8
(Libby's) whole kernel	½ cup	16.0
(Stokely-Van Camp)	½ cup	17.5
Frozen (Birds Eye)	⅓ of pkg.	17.0
SUGAR:		
Brown	1 T.	12.5
Confectioners'	1 T.	7.7
Granulated	1 T.	11.9
Maple	1¾" x 1¼" x ½" piece	27.0
SUGAR CORN POPS, cereal		
(Kellogg's)	1 cup	26.0
SUGAR CRISP, cereal (Post)	⅞ cup	25.5
SUGAR PUFFS, cereal		
(Malt-O-Meal)	⅞ cup	26.0
SUGAR SMACKS, cereal (Kellogg's)	¾ cup	25.0
SUGAR SUBSTITUTE:		
(Featherweight) liquid or tablet	Any quantity	0.
Sprinkle Sweet (Pillsbury)	⅛ tsp.	.5
Sugar-Like (Dia-Mel)	1 packet	1.0
(S&W) Nutradiet	1 tsp.	0.
Sweet'n-it (Dia-Mel) liquid	5 drops	0.
Sweet*10 (Pillsbury)	⅛ tsp.	0.
(Weight Watchers)	1 packet	1.0
*SUKIYAKI DINNER, frozen		
(Chun King) stir fry	⅙ of pkg.	3.0
SUNFLOWER SEED (Fisher):		
In hull, roasted, salted	1 oz.	3.0
Hulled, dry or oil roasted, salted	1 oz.	5.6
SUZY Q (Hostess):		
Banana	1 cake	38.4
Chocolate	1 cake	36.4
SWEETBREADS, calf, braised	4 oz.	0.
SWEET POTATO:		
Fresh, baked, peeled	5" x 1" potato	35.8
Canned, heavy syrup	4-oz. serving	31.2
Frozen:		
(Green Giant) glazed	⅓ of pkg.	22.7

Food and Description	Measure or Quantity	Carbohydrates (grams)
(Mrs. Paul's) candied, with apple	4-oz. serving	36.1
*SWEET & SOUR DINNER (Chun King) stir fry	⅛ of pkg.	10.0
SWEET & SOUR ORIENTAL, canned (La Choy):		
Chicken	7½-oz. serving	50.0
Pork	7½-oz. serving	48.0
SWEET & SOUR PORK, frozen (Chun King)	½ of 12-oz. pouch	22.0
SWISS STEAK, frozen (Swanson) *TV Brand*	10-oz. dinner	40.0
SWORDFISH, broiled	3" x 3" x ½" steak	0.
SYRUP:		
Sweetened:		
Apricot (Smucker's)	1 T.	13.0
Blackberry (Smucker's)	1 T.	13.0
Blueberry (Smucker's)	1 T.	13.0
Boysenberry (Smucker's)	1 T.	13.0
Chocolate or chocolate flavored:		
Bosco	1 T.	13.3
(Hershey's)	1 T. (.7 oz.)	11.7
Milk Mate	1½ T.	18.0
Corn, *Karo*, dark or light	1 T.	14.6
Cane	1 T.	14.0
Maple, *Karo*, imitation	1 T.	14.2
Pancake or waffle:		
Golden Griddle	1 T.	13.4
Karo	1 T.	14.4
Log Cabin	1 T.	13.1
Mrs. Butterworth's	1 T.	13.0
Raspberry (Smucker's)	1 T.	11.6
Strawberry (Smucker's)	1 T.	13.0
Dietetic:		
Blueberry (Featherweight)	1 T.	3.0
Chocolate flavored:		
(Dia-Mel)	1 T.	3.3
(Featherweight)	1 T.	7.0
Chocolate flavored:		
(No-Cal)	1 T.	0.
Coffee (No-Cal)	1 T.	1.2
Cola (No-Cal)	1 T.	Tr.
Maple, imitation (S&W) *Nutradiet*	1 T.	3.0
Pancake or waffle:		
(Aunt Jemima)	1 T.	7.3
(Diet Delight)	1 T.	4.0
(Tillie Lewis) *Tasti-Diet*	1 T.	1.0

Food and Description	Measure or Quantity	Carbohydrates (grams)

T

TACO:
*(Ortega)	1 taco	15.0
*Mix (Durkee)	½ cup	3.8
Shell (Ortega)	.4-oz. shell	7.7
TACO SEASONING MIX (French's)	1¼-oz. pkg.	16.0

TAMALE:
Canned:
(Hormel) beef, *Short Orders*	7½-oz. can	17.0
(Nalley's) beef	8-oz. serving	25.0
Old El Paso, with chili gravy	1 tamale	11.5
Frozen (Hormel) beef	1 tamale	11.3
TAMALE PIE (Nalley's)	4-oz. serving	12.5
TANG, grape or orange	½ cup	15.0

TANGERINE or MANDARIN ORANGE:
Fresh (Sunkist)	1 large tangerine	10.0
Canned, regular pack (Del Monte) solids & liq.	¼ of 22-oz. can	25.3
Canned, dietetic pack, solids & liq.:		
(Diet Delight) juice pack	½ cup	13.0
(Featherweight) water pack	½ cup	8.0
(S&W) *Nutradiet*	½ cup	7.0
TANGERINE DRINK, canned (Hi-C)	6 fl. oz.	23.0
*TANGERINE JUICE, frozen (Minute Maid)	6 fl. oz.	20.8
TARRAGON (French's)	1 tsp.	.7
TASTEEOS, cereal (Ralston Purina)	1¼ cups	22.0

TEA (Lipton):
Bag:
Regular	1 bag	0.
Flavored:		
Black Rum, Mint or Quietly Chamomile	1 bag	<1.0
Almond Pleasure or Cinnamon Apple	1 bag	0.
*Instant:		
Lemon flavored	8 fl. oz.	1.0
100%	8 fl. oz.	0.
TEAM, cereal	1 cup	24.0

TEA MIX, ICED:
*(Lipton) lemon-flavored with sugar	8 fl. oz.	16.0
*Nestea, lemon-flavored	8 fl. oz.	.2

Food and Description	Measure or Quantity	Carbohydrates (grams)
TERIYAKI, frozen (Stouffer's) beef, with rice & vegetables	10-oz. serving	40.9
TEQUILA SUNRISE COCKTAIL, canned (Mr. Boston) 12½% alcohol	3 fl. oz.	14.4
*TEXTURED VEGETABLE PROTEIN (Morningstar Farms):		
Breakfast link	1 link	.3
Breakfast patties	1 patty	3.2
Breakfast strips	1 strip	.2
Grillers	1 piece	4.5
THUNDERBIRD WINE (Gallo):		
14% alcohol	3 fl. oz.	8.1
20% alcohol	3 fl. oz.	7.5
THURINGER:		
(Best's Kosher; Osherwitz)	1-oz. serving	.3
(Hormel):		
Buffet	1-oz. serving	.3
Old Smokehouse	1-oz. serving	.1
Summer sausage	1-oz. slice	.2
(Louis Rich) turkey	1-oz. serving	<1.0
(Oscar Mayer):		
Summer sausage	1-oz. slice	.3
Summer sausage, beef	8-oz. slice	.7
THYME, dried (French's)	1 tsp.	1.0
TIA MARIA (Hiram Walker)	1 fl. oz.	10.0
TIGER TAILS (Hostess)	1 piece	38.1
TOASTER CAKE or PASTRY:		
Flavor Kist (Schulze and Burch):		
Regular	1 pastry	35.0
Frosted:		
All flavors except fudge	1 pastry	36.0
Fudge	1 pastry	34.0
Pop Tarts (Kellogg's):		
Regular:		
Blueberry or cherry	1 pastry	36.0
Brown sugar cinnamon	1 pastry	33.0
Chocolate chip	1 pastry	34.0
Strawberry	1 pastry	37.0
Frosted:		
Blueberry or strawberry	1 pastry	38.0
Brown sugar-cinnamon	1 pastry	34.0
Cherry or chocolate-vanilla creme	1 pastry	37.0
Chocolate fudge, concord grape, dutch apple or raspberry	1 pastry	36.0
Toastettes (Nabisco) all flavors	1 pastry	35.0

Food and Description	Measure or Quantity	Carbohydrates (grams)
Toast-R-Cake (Thomas'):		
Blueberry	1 cake	17.7
Bran	1 cake	19.9
Corn	1 cake	18.7
TOASTY O's, cereal (Malt-O-Meal)	1¼ cups	20.0
TOMATO:		
Fresh, cherry, whole	4 pieces	3.2
Fresh, regular, whole	1 med.	7.0
Canned, regular pack:		
(Contadina) sliced	4-oz. serving	8.5
(Stokely-Van Camp) stewed	½ cup	7.5
(Van Camp) whole	½ cup	5.0
Canned, dietetic pack:		
(Diet Delight)	½ cup	5.0
(Featherweight)	½ cup	4.0
(S&W) *Nutradiet*, whole	½ cup	5.0
TOMATO JUICE:		
Canned, regular pack:		
(Campbell)	6 fl. oz.	8.0
(Del Monte)	6 fl. oz.	7.4
(Libby's)	6 fl. oz.	7.5
Musselman's	6 fl. oz.	7.0
Canned, dietetic pack:		
(Diet Delight)	6 fl. oz.	7.0
(Featherweight)	6 fl. oz.	7.5
(S&W) *Nutradiet*	6 fl. oz.	8.0
TOMATO JUICE COCKTAIL, canned:		
(Ocean Spray) *Firehouse Jubilee*	6 fl. oz.	9.1
Snap-E-Tom	6 fl. oz.	7.0
TOMATO PASTE:		
Canned, regular pack:		
(Del Monte)	6-oz. can	33.8
(Hunt's)	6-oz. can	30.0
Canned, dietetic pack (Featherweight)	6-oz. can	35.0
TOMATO & PEPPER, HOT CHILI		
(Ortega) Jalapeno	1-oz. serving	1.0
TOMATO, PICKLED (Claussen), green, halves, kosher	1-oz. piece	1.1
TOMATO PUREE, canned:		
Regular (Contadina) heavy	1 cup	26.4
Dietetic (Featherweight)	1 cup	20.0
TOMATO SAUCE, canned:		
(Contadina)	1 cup	19.6
(Del Monte):		
Regular	1 cup	17.0
Hot	1 cup	8.5

134

Food and Description	Measure or Quantity	Carbohydrates (grams)
With mushroom	1 cup	21.4
With onion	1 cup	23.0
With tomato tidbits	1 cup	5.7
(Hunt's)		
Regular	4-oz. serving	8.0
With bits	4-oz. serving	8.0
With herbs	4-oz. serving	12.0
With mushrooms	4-oz. serving	9.0
Prima Salsa	4-oz. serving	20.0
(Libby's)	4-oz. serving	9.8
TOMATO SOUP, canned:		
Regular pack:		
*(Campbell):		
Regular, made with milk	10-oz. serving	27.0
Regular, made with water	10-oz. serving	20.0
With rice, old fashioned	11-oz. serving	29.0
*(Rokeach):		
Made with milk	10-oz. serving	27.0
Made with water	10-oz. serving	20.0
Dietetic pack:		
(Campbell) low sodium	7¼-oz. can	22.0
*(Dia-Mel)	8-oz. serving	11.0
*TOMATO SOUP MIX (Lipton):		
Cup-A-Soup	6 fl. oz.	17.0
TOM COLLINS:		
Canned (Mr. Boston) 12½% alcohol	3 fl. oz.	10.8
Mix, dry (Holland House)	1 serving	17.0
TONGUE, beef, braised	4-oz. serving	.5
TOPPING:		
Regular:		
Butterscotch (Smucker's)	1 T.	16.5
Caramel (Smucker's)	1 T.	16.5
Chocolate fudge (Hershey's)	1 T.	9.3
Peanut butter caramel		
(Smucker's)	1 T.	14.5
Pecans in syrup (Smucker's)	1 T.	14.0
Pineapple (Smucker's)	1 T.	16.0
TOPPING:		
Dietetic, chocolate (Diet Delight)	1 T.	3.6
TOPPING, WHIPPED:		
Regular:		
Cool Whip (Birds Eye)	1 T.	1.3
Lucky Whip, aerosol	1 T.	.5
Whip Topping (Rich's)	¼ oz.	1.2
Dietetic (Featherweight)	1 T.	.5
*TOPPING, WHIPPED, MIX:		
(Dream Whip)	1 T.	1.0
Dietetic (D-Zerta)	1 T.	0.

Food and Description	Measure or Quantity	Carbohydrates (grams)
TOP RAMEN (Nissin Foods) beef	3-oz. serving	50.5
TORTILLA (Amigos)	6" x ⅛" tortilla	19.7
TOSTADA SHELL (Ortega)	1 shell	6.0
TOTAL, cereal (General Mills)	1 cup	23.0
TRIPE, canned (Libby's)	6-oz. serving	1.1
TRIPLE SEC LIQUEUR:		
(Bols)	1 fl. oz.	8.8
(Mr. Boston)	1 fl. oz.	8.5
TRIX, cereal (General Mills)	1 cup	25.0
TUNA:		
Canned in oil:		
(Breast O' Chicken) solids & liq.	6½-oz. can	0.
(Chicken of the Sea) chunk, light, solids & liq.	6½-oz. can	Tr.
(Star-Kist) solid, white, solids & liq.	7-oz. serving	0.
Canned in water:		
(Breast O' Chicken)	6½-oz. can	0.
(Chicken of the Sea) white	7-oz. can	1.0
(Featherweight)	6½-oz. can	0.
TUNA HELPER (General Mills):		
Cheese sauce	⅕ of pkg.	28.0
Country dumplings or creamy noodles	⅕ of pkg.	31.0
TUNA NOODLES CASSEROLE, frozen (Stouffer's)	5¾-oz. serving	18.0
TUNA & PEAS, frozen (Green Giant) creamed	5-oz. serving	9.8
TUNA PIE, frozen:		
(Banquet)	8-oz. pie	42.7
(Morton)	8-oz. pie	36.4
TUNA SALAD:		
Home recipe	4-oz. serving	4.0
Canned (Carnation)	1½-oz. serving	3.2
TURBOT MEAL, frozen (Weight Watchers):		
Regular	8-oz. meal	12.0
Stuffed	16-oz. meal	25.9
TURKEY:		
Barbecued (Louis Rich) breast, half	1 oz.	0.
Canned:		
(Hormel) chunk	6¾-oz. serving	.6
(Swanson) chunk	2½-oz. serving	0.
Packaged:		
(Eckrich) sliced	1-oz. serving	1.3
(Hormel) breast	.8-oz. slice	.1

Food and Description	Measure or Quantity	Carbohydrates (grams)
(Louis Rich):		
Turkey bologna	1-oz. slice	1.0
Turkey cotto salami	1-oz. slice	<1.0
Turkey pastrami	1-oz. serving	<1.0
(Oscar Mayer) breast meat	.8-oz. slice	0.
Roasted:		
Flesh & skin	4-oz. serving	0.
Dark meat	2½" x 1⅝" x ¼" slice	0.
Light meat	4" x 2" x ¼" slice	0.
Smoked (Louis Rich):		
Drumsticks	1 oz. (without bone)	<1.0
Wing drumettes	1 oz. (without bone)	<1.0
TURKEY DINNER or ENTREE,		
frozen:		
(Banquet):		
Regular	11-oz. dinner	27.8
Man Pleaser	19-oz. dinner	73.8
(Morton):		
Country Table, sliced	15-oz. dinner	81.1
King Size	19-oz. dinner	64.8
(Swanson):		
With gravy & dressing	9¼-oz. entree	21.0
Hungry Man	19-oz. dinner	81.0
Hungry Man	13¼-oz. entree	34.0
TV Brand	11½-oz. dinner	45.0
(Weight Watchers) sliced, 3-compartment	15¼-oz. meal	37.3
TURKEY PIE, frozen:		
(Banquet)	8-oz. pie	40.6
(Morton)	8-oz. pie	31.8
(Stouffer's)	10-oz. pie	34.7
(Swanson):		
Regular	8-oz. pie	47.0
Hungry Man	1-lb. pie	64.0
TURKEY SALAD, canned		
(Carnation) *Spreadable*	1½-oz. serving	3.0
TURKEY SOUP, canned:		
Regular pack:		
*(Ann Page) & noodle	1 cup	17.8
(Campbell):		
Chunky	18½-oz. can	30.0
*Condensed, noodle	10-oz. serving	10.0
*Condensed, vegetable	10-oz. serving	10.0
Dietetic pack (Campbell) low sodium, & noodle	7½-oz. can	7.0
TURKEY TETRAZZINI, frozen:		
(Stouffer's)	6-oz. serving	16.9
(Weight Watchers)	13-oz. bag	36.9

137

Food and Description	Measure or Quantity	Carbohydrates (grams)
TURMERIC (French's)	1 tsp.	1.3
TURNIP:		
Boiled, drained, diced	½ cup	3.8
Boiled, drained, mashed	½ cup	5.6
TURNIP GREENS:		
Canned (Sunshine) chopped, solids & liq.	½ cup	2.5
Frozen:		
(Birds Eye)	⅓ of pkg.	3.0
(Seabrook Farms) chopped	⅓ of pkg.	3.4
(Southland) chopped	⅕ of 16-oz. pkg.	4.0
TURNOVER:		
Frozen (Pepperidge Farm):		
Apple or cherry	1 turnover	30.0
Blueberry	1 turnover	32.0
Peach	1 turnover	33.0
Raspberry	1 turnover	37.0
Refrigerated (Pillsbury):		
Apple	1 turnover	23.0
Blueberry	1 turnover	22.0
Cherry	1 turnover	24.0
TWINKIE (Hostess):		
Regular	1 cake	26.1
Devil's food	1 cake	24.7

V

Food and Description	Measure or Quantity	Carbohydrates (grams)
VALPOLICELLA WINE (Antinori)	3 fl. oz.	6.3
VANDERMINT, liqueur	1 fl. oz.	10.2
VANILLA EXTRACT (Virginia Dare)	1 tsp.	Tr.
VANILLA ICE CREAM:		
(Baskin-Robbins):		
Regular	1 scoop (2½ fl. oz.)	15.6
French	1 scoop (2½ fl. oz.)	15.9
Good Humor	4 fl. oz.	14.0
(Meadow Gold)	¼ pt.	16.0
VEAL	Any quantity	0.
VEAL DINNER, frozen:		
(Banquet) parmigian:		
Buffet Supper	2-lb. pkg.	119.1
Dinner	11-oz. dinner	42.1
(Green Giant) breaded, parmigiana	14-oz. serving	36.6
(Morton) parmigiana	11-oz. dinner	28.1
(Swanson) parmigiana:		
Hungry Man	20½-oz. dinner	75.0

Food and Description	Measure or Quantity	Carbohydrates (grams)
TV Brand	12½-oz. dinner	51.0
(Weight Watchers) parmigiana, 2-compartment	9-oz. meal	12.0
VEAL STEAK, frozen (Hormel):		
Regular	4-oz. serving	2.1
Breaded	4-oz. serving	13.1
V-8 (See VEGETABLE JUICE COCKTAIL)		
VEGETABLE FLAKES (French's) dehydrated	1 T.	3.0
VEGETABLE JUICE COCKTAIL, canned:		
Regular pack:		
V-8:		
Regular	6 fl. oz.	8.0
Spicy hot	6 fl. oz.	8.0
Dietetic:		
(S&W) *Nutradiet,* low sodium	6 fl. oz.	8.0
V-8, low sodium	6 fl. oz.	8.0
VEGETABLES, MIXED:		
Canned, regular pack:		
(Chun King) chow mein, solids & liq.	4-oz. serving	2.0
(Del Monte) drained	½ cup	7.4
(La Choy):		
Chinese	1 cup	1.6
Chop suey	1 cup	6.9
(Libby's) solids & liq.	½ cup	9.8
(Stokely-Van Camp) solids & liq.	½ cup	8.5
Canned, dietetic pack (Featherweight) low sodium	½ cup	8.0
Frozen:		
(Birds Eye):		
Americana Recipe:		
New England style	⅓ of pkg.	11.7
New Orleans style	⅓ of pkg.	13.8
San Francisco style	⅓ of pkg.	6.4
International Recipe:		
Chinese style	⅓ of pkg.	10.2
Hawaiian style	⅓ of pkg.	12.0
Italian style	⅓ of pkg.	8.3
Japanese style	⅓ of pkg.	9.1
Stir Fry:		
Chinese style	⅓ of pkg.	7.0
Mandarin style	⅓ of pkg.	6.0
(Green Giant):		
Chinese style	½ cup	10.0
Hawaiian style	½ cup	16.5

Food and Description	Measure or Quantity	Carbohydrates (grams)
Mixed	½ cup	8.0
(Kounty Kist)	½ cup	8.0
(La Choy):		
Chinese	5-oz. serving	5.3
Japanese	5-oz. serving	5.8
(Southland):		
California blend	⅕ of 16-oz. pkg.	7.0
Gumbo	⅕ of 16-oz. pkg.	10.0
Stew	4 oz.	14.0
VEGETABLE SOUP, canned:		
Regular pack:		
(Campbell):		
Chunky:		
Regular	10¾-oz. can	24.0
Beef, old fashioned	19-oz. can	38.0
*Condensed:		
Regular	10-oz. serving	16.0
Beef	10-oz. serving	10.0
Old fashioned	10-oz. serving	12.0
Vegetarian	10-oz. serving	14.0
*Semi-condensed, *Soup For One:*		
Beef, burly	7¾-oz. can	19.0
Old world	7¾-oz. can	18.0
*(Rokeach) vegetarian	10-oz. serving	15.0
Canned, dietetic pack:		
(Campbell):		
Regular, low sodium	7¼-oz. can	14.0
Beef, low sodium	7⅓-oz. can	8.0
*(Dia-Mel):		
Regular	8-oz. serving	12.0
& beef	8-oz. serving	11.0
*Frozen (Mother's Own)	8-oz. serving	<1.0
*VEGETABLE SOUP MIX (Lipton):		
Beef	8 fl. oz.	7.0
Beef, *Cup-A-Soup*	6 fl. oz.	8.0
Harvest Country style, *Cup-A-Soup*	6 fl. oz.	20.0
Spring, *Cup-A-Soup*	1 fl. oz.	7.0
VEGETABLE STEW, canned, *Dinty Moore*	7½-oz. serving	18.3
"VEGETARIAN FOODS":		
Canned or dry:		
Chicken, fried (Loma Linda) with gravy	1½-oz. piece	1.9
Chili (Worthington)	5-oz. serving	20.0
Choplet (Worthington)	1 choplet	3.0
Cutlet (Worthington)	1 slice	2.6

Food and Description	Measure or Quantity	Carbohydrates (grams)
Dinner cuts (Loma Linda) drained	1 cut	1.6
Franks, big (Loma Linda)	1.9-oz. frank	4.1
FriChik (Worthington)	1 piece	1.0
Granburger (Worthington)	6 T.	12.0
Linketts (Loma Linda) drained	1.3-oz. link	2.2
Little links (Loma Linda) drained	.8-oz. link	1.3
Non-meatballs (Worthington)	1 meatball	2.3
Nuteena (Loma Linda)	½" slice	7.6
Proteena (Loma Linda)	½" slice	6.5
Redi-burger (Loma Linda)	½" slice	8.8
Sandwich spread (Loma Linda)	1 T.	1.7
Savorex (Loma Linda)	1 T.	2.0
Soyagen, all purpose powder (Loma Linda)	1 T.	4.7
Soyalac (Loma Linda):		
I-Soyalac	1 cup	17.0
Concentrate, liquid	1 cup	33.8
Ready to use	1 cup	15.9
Soyameat (Worthington):		
Sliced beef	1 slice	1.5
Diced chicken	¼ cup	2.0
Sliced chicken	1 slice	1.0
Salisbury steak	1 slice	2.0
Soyamel, any kind (Worthington)	1 oz.	15.2
Stew pac (Loma Linda) drained	1 piece	.6
Super links (Worthington)	1 link	4.0
Swiss steak with gravy (Loma Linda)	1 steak	8.9
Vega-links (Worthington)	1 link	6.0
Vege-burger (Loma Linda)	½ cup	4.3
Vege-burger (Loma Linda) no salt added	½ cup	6.9
Vegelona (Loma Linda)	½" slice	7.0
Wheat protein	4 oz.	10.0
Wheat protein, nuts or peanuts	4 oz.	20.1
Wheat and soy protein, soy or other vegetable oil	4 oz.	10.9
Worthington 209	1 slice	1.5
Frozen:		
Beef-like roll (Worthington)	1 slice	4.0
Beef pie (Worthington)	1 pie	51.0
Bologna (Loma Linda)	1 oz.	2.8
Chicken (Loma Linda)	1-oz. slice	1.5
Chicken pie (Worthington)	1 pie	42.0
Chic-Ketts (Worthington)	½ cup	6.0
FriPats (Worthington)	1 pat	3.0

Food and Description	Measure or Quantity	Carbohydrates (grams)
Meatballs (Loma Linda)	1 meatball	2.2
Prosage (Worthington)	1 link	1.7
Roast beef (Loma Linda)	1 oz.	1.3
Salami (Loma Linda)	1-oz. slice	1.7
Sausage, breakfast (Loma Linda)	1-oz. slice	1.4
Sizzle burger (Loma Linda)	2½-oz. burger	13.3
Stripples (Worthington)	1 slice	.8
Turkey (Loma Linda)	1-oz. slice	1.6
Wham (Worthington) roll	2½ oz.	4.0
VERMOUTH:		
Dry & extra dry (Lejon)	1 fl. oz.	1.1
Sweet (Taylor)	1 fl. oz.	3.8
VICHYSSOISE SOUP (Crosse & Blackwell), cream of	6½-oz. serving	5.0
VIENNA SAUSAGE:		
(Hormel):		
Regular	1 sausage	Tr.
Chicken	1-oz. serving	.2
(Libby's):		
With barbecue sauce	.7-oz. sausage	.5
With beef broth	.7-oz. sausage	.2
VINEGAR, red or white wine (Regina)	1 T.	Tr.

W

WAFFELOS, cereal (Ralston	1 cup	25.0
WAFFLE, frozen:		
(Aunt Jemima) jumbo	1 waffle	14.5
(Eggo):		
Blueberry or strawberry	1 waffle	18.0
Home style	1 waffle	17.0
(Roman Meal):		
Regular	1 waffle	16.5
Golden Delight	1 waffle	15.1
WALLBANGER COCKTAIL, canned (Mr. Boston) 12½% alcohol	3 fl. oz.	9.6
WALNUT, English or Persian (Diamond A)	1 cup	12.8
WATER CHESTNUT, canned:		
(Chun King) solids & liq.	8½-oz. can	22.0
(La Choy) drained	¼ of 8-oz. can	3.9
WATERCRESS	½ cup	.5
WATERMELON:		
Wedge	4″ x 8″ wedge	27.3
Diced	½ cup	5.1

Food and Description	Measure or Quantity	Carbohydrates (grams)
WELSH RAREBIT:		
Home recipe	1 cup	14.6
Frozen:		
(Green Giant)	5-oz. serving	11.4
(Stouffer's)	5-oz. serving	16.9
WESTERN DINNER, frozen:		
(Banquet)	11-oz. dinner	32.4
(Morton) *Round-Up*	11.8-oz. dinner	33.5
(Swanson):		
Hungry Man	17¾-oz. dinner	70.0
TV Brand	11¾-oz. dinner	42.0
WHEAT FLAKES CEREAL:		
(Breakfast Best)	1 cup	30.3
(Van Brode)	¾ cup	22.7
WHEAT GERM, raw (Elam's)	1 oz.	12.8
WHEAT GERM CEREAL:		
(Kellogg's) all flavors	¼ cup	13.0
(Kretschmer):		
Regular	¼ cup	8.8
With brown sugar & honey	¼ cup	17.0
WHEATIES, cereal (General Mills)	1 cup	23.0
WHEAT & OATMEAL, cereal, hot		
(Elam's)	1 oz.	18.8
WHEAT & RAISIN CHEX, cereal		
(Ralston Purina)	¾ cup	30.0
WHISKEY SOUR COCKTAIL,		
canned (Mr. Boston) 12½% alcohol	3 fl. oz.	14.4
WHITEFISH, LAKE:		
Baked, stuffed	4-oz. serving	6.6
Smoked	4-oz. serving	0.
WIENER WRAP, refrigerated		
(Pillsbury) plain or cheese	1 wrap	10.0
WILD BERRY DRINK (Hi-C)	6 fl. oz.	22.0
WINE, COOKING (Regina):		
Burgundy	¼ cup	1.0
Sauterne	¼ cup	.5
Sherry	¼ cup	5.0
*WON TON SOUP:		
*Canned (Campbell)	10-oz. serving	6.0
*Frozen (La Choy)	1 cup	12.3

Y

YEAST, BAKER'S (Fleischmann's):		
Dry, active	¼ oz.	3.0
Fresh & household, active	.6-oz. cake	2.0

Food and Description	Measure or Quantity	Carbohydrates (grams)
YOGURT:		
Regular:		
Plain:		
(Bison)	8-oz. container	16.8
(Colombo) *Natural Light*	8-oz. container	17.0
(Dannon)	8-oz. container	17.0
(Friendship)	8-oz. container	15.0
(Sweet 'n Low)	8-oz. container	15.0
Yoplait (General Mills)	6-oz. container	14.0
Apple:		
(Bison) dutch	8-oz. container	45.9
(Colombo) spiced	8-oz. container	39.0
(Dannon) dutch	8-oz. container	49.0
Mélangé (Dannon)	6-oz. container	31.0
(New Country) crisp	8-oz. container	42.0
(Sweet 'n Low) dutch	8-oz. container	33.0
Apricot:		
(Bison)	8-oz. container	45.9
(Dannon)	8-oz. container	49.0
Banana:		
(Dannon)	8-oz. container	49.0
LeShake (Kellogg)	8-oz. container	28.0
Banana-strawberry (Colombo)	8-oz. container	38.0
Blueberry:		
(Bison)	8-oz. container	45.9
(Colombo)	8-oz. container	38.0
(Dannon)	8-oz. container	49.0
(Friendship)	8-oz. container	57.0
Mélangé (Dannon)	6-oz. container	31.0
(Sweet 'n Low)	8-oz. container	33.0
Yoplait (General Mills)	6-oz. container	32.0
Boysenberry:		
(Bison)	8-oz. container	45.9
(Dannon)	8-oz. container	49.0
(Sweet 'n Low)	8-oz. container	33.0
Cherry:		
(Bison):		
Regular	8-oz. container	45.9
Light	6-oz. container	28.1
(Colombo)	8-oz. container	34.0
(Dannon)	8-oz. container	49.0
(Friendship)	8-oz. container	57.0
Mélangé (Dannon)	6-oz. container	31.0
(New Country) supreme	8-oz. container	44.0
(Sweet 'n Low)	8-oz. container	33.0
Yoplait (General Mills)	6-oz. container	32.0
Cherry-vanilla (Colombo)	8-oz. container	40.0

Food and Description	Measure or Quantity	Carbohydrates (grams)
Coffee:		
(Colombo)	8-oz. container	29.0
(Dannon)	8-oz. container	32.0
Date-walnut-raisin (Bison)	8-oz. container	45.9
Naja (Alta-Dena Dairy)	1 container	40.0
Fruit crunch (New Country)	8-oz. container	42.0
Granola strawberry (Colombo)	8-oz. container	40.0
Guava (Colombo)	8-oz. container	40.0
Hawaiian salad (New Country)	8-oz. container	42.0
Honey 'n Berries (New Country)	8-oz. container	43.0
Honey vanilla (Colombo)	8-oz. container	30.0
Lemon:		
(Dannon)	8-oz. container	32.0
(New Country) ripple	8-oz. container	43.0
(Sweet 'n Low)	8-oz. container	33.0
Yoplait (General Mills)	6-oz. container	32.0
Orange, Yoplait (General Mills)	6-oz. container	32.0
Orange supreme (New Country)	8-oz. container	43.0
Peach:		
(Bison)	8-oz. container	45.9
(Dannon)	8-oz. container	49.0
(Friendship)	8-oz. container	57.0
(New Country) 'n cream	8-oz. container	43.0
(Sweet 'n Low)	8-oz. container	33.0
Peach melba (Colombo)	8-oz. container	37.0
Piña Colada:		
(Colombo)	8-oz. container	40.0
(Dannon)	8-oz. container	49.0
Pineapple:		
(Bison) light	6-oz. container	28.1
Mélangé (Dannon)	6-oz. container	31.0
Pineapple-orange (Dannon)	8-oz. container	49.0
Raspberry:		
(Bison)	8-oz. container	45.9
(Dannon) red	8-oz. container	49.0
(Friendship)	8-oz. container	57.0
LeShake (Kellogg)	8-oz. container	29.0
Mélangé (Dannon)	6-oz. container	31.0
(Sweet 'n Low)	8-oz. container	33.0
Strawberry:		
(Bison) light	6-oz. container	28.1
(Colombo)	8-oz. container	36.0
(Friendship)	8-oz. container	57.0
LeShake (Kellogg)	8-oz. container	27.0
Mélangé (Dannon)	6-oz. container	31.0
(New Country) supreme	8-oz. container	43.0
(Sweet 'n Low)	8-oz. container	33.0

Food and Description	Measure or Quantity	Carbohydrates (grams)
Strawberry banana (Sweet 'n Low)	8-oz. container	33.0
Strawberry colada (Colombo)	8-oz. container	36.0
Tropical fruit (Sweet 'n Low)	8-oz. container	33.0
Vanilla:		
(Dannon)	8-oz. container	32.0
LeShake (Kellogg)	8-oz. container	32.0
Frozen, hard:		
Banana (Dannon):		
Danny-Yo	3½-oz. serving	21.0
Danny-in-a-Cup	8-oz. cup	42.0
Boysenberry (Dannon):		
Danny-On-A-Stick, carob coated	2½-fl.-oz. bar	13.0
Danny-Yo	3½-oz. serving	21.0
Boysenberry-swirl (Bison)	¼ of 16-oz. container	24.0
Cherry-vanilla (Bison)	¼ of 16-oz. container	24.0
Chocolate:		
(Bison)	¼ of 16-oz. container	24.0
(Colombo) bar, chocolate-covered	1 bar	17.0
(Dannon):		
Danny-in-a-Cup	8-fl.-oz. cup	42.0
Danny-On-A-Stick, chocolate-covered	2½-fl.-oz. bar	13.0
Chocolate chip (Bison)	¼ of 16-oz. container	24.0
Chocolate, chocolate chip (Colombo)	4-oz. serving	28.0
Mocha (Colombo)	1 bar	14.0
Piña Colada:		
(Colombo)	4-oz. serving	20.0
(Dannon):		
Danny-in-a-Cup	8-oz. cup	42.0
Danny-On-A-Stick	2½-fl.-oz. bar	13.0
Raspberry swirl (Bison)	¼ of 16-oz. container	24.0
Strawberry:		
(Bison)	¼ of 16-oz. container	24.0
(Colombo)	4-oz. serving	20.0
(Dannon):		
Danny-in-a-Cup	8-oz. cup	42.0
Danny-On-A-Stick, chocolate coated	2½-fl.-oz. bar	13.0
Vanilla:		
(Bison)	¼ of 16-oz. container	24.0
(Colombo):		
Regular	4-oz. serving	20.0
Bar, chocolate covered	1 bar	17.0

Food and Description	Measure or Quantity	Carbohydrates (grams)
(Dannon):		
Danny-On-A-Stick,		
uncoated	2½-fl.-oz. bar	13.0
Danny-Yo	3½-oz. serving	21.0
Frozen, soft (Colombo) all flavors	6-fl.-oz. serving	24.0

Z

ZINFANDEL WINE (Inglenook)		
Vintage	3 fl. oz.	.3
ZITI, frozen (Weight Watchers)	12½-oz. meal	41.2
ZWIEBACK (Gerber; Nabisco)	1 piece	5.0

Other SIGNET Books of Special Interest